Multidisciplinary Management
of Prostate Cancer

Vincenzo Gentile • Valeria Panebianco •
Alessandro Sciarra

Editors

Multidisciplinary Management of Prostate Cancer

The Role of the Prostate Cancer Unit

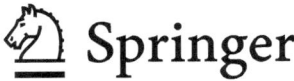 Springer

Editors
Vincenzo Gentile
Alessandro Sciarra
Department of Urology
Sapienza University
Rome, Italy

Valeria Panebianco
Department of Radiological Sciences
Oncology & Pathology
Sapienza University, Policlinico Umberto I
Rome, Italy

ISBN 978-3-319-04384-5   ISBN 978-3-319-04385-2 (eBook)
DOI 10.1007/978-3-319-04385-2
Springer Cham Heidelberg New York Dordrecht London

Library of Congress Control Number: 2014934693

Printed on acid-free paper

Springer is part of Springer Science+Business Media (www.springer.com)

In memory of Franco Di Silverio

Foreword

Patient-centred care features high on political agendas nowadays which is also reflected in a concept such as personalised medicine which has been introduced fairly recently. The aim is to provide the best care for an individual patient, taking into account a patient's personal circumstance and preferences, and facilitate the involvement of patients in their own health-care needs. It is in this setting that multidisciplinary team (MDT) management of patients should be viewed. Multidisciplinary care, involving clinicians from all related specialties in the treatment of a disease, is not a new notion, but the effective implementation of MDT approaches is much more recent, where considerable differences are seen between countries and for different pathologies. Uptake will also be greatly affected by a number of variables such as organisation of health-care systems, as well as on the type and size of health-care facilities.

Whilst multidisciplinary care will be most relevant in all settings, major impact is found in cancer care, possibly because the stakes are perceived to be higher. This publication addresses the many aspects of MDT processes in patients suspected of harbouring prostate cancer and their treatment. Prostate cancer is the most common cancer in elderly males in Europe, and with the proportion of elderly men in the general population increasing, as well as life expectancy, this translates directly into a higher claim on professional care.

The authors of this publication very convincingly argue that within an MDT setting, the time between diagnosis and treatment is shorter, resulting in improved outcomes as compared to non-MDT approaches. Secondary benefit is that less time spent in the health-care system will be a costing benefit for the community. Also, MDT approaches have a distinct effect on the treatment modalities offered to patients, by reducing the physician bias in the selection of management strategies. The increasing complexity of the many treatment options that are potentially available for prostate cancer care will promote involvement of super-specialists and this is where an MDT setting will obviously offer considerable gain. Prostate cancer management is a field where more and more new diagnostic and treatment modalities are emerging: technological (improved imaging techniques, minimally invasive technologies) as well as drug therapies. It is most interesting that in some chapters, the authors provide data gathered from studies conducted at their own units. This information—as well as literature identified though what seems to be a very sound assessment of the available data—support their case when comparing

MDT outcomes to non-MDT data. This is clearly a most compelling approach to support their arguments; i.e. MDT management will improve cancer outcomes and support the role of the patient as an active and informed partner in his journey through the health-care system.

Evidence-based health-care provision, underpinning MDT approaches, is clearly not at odds with the concept of patient-centred care as shown by the data presented in this book. Having access to a complete team of medical specialists will only allow for optimising treatment choices, fully respecting individual patients needs and personal circumstances.

But, the title of this publication is somewhat deceptive. This book, in fact, provides a 360° view of prostate cancer management. Even for those readers first and foremost interested in prostate cancer management and to a lesser degree in organisational matters, this book will certainly provide a most comprehensive update. For many clinicians MDT management of prostate cancer will be a given, but it is still extremely gratifying to see that the available data show clear benefits. MDT management will offer inter-organisational safeguards and enhance the care for our patients diagnosed with prostate cancer. I most certainly should like to commend the authors for making such a compelling case for this approach.

Malmö, Sweden   Per-Anders Abrahamsson

Contents

Michele Innocenzi and Giuseppe D'Eramo

1.1   Introduction

Oncology care has rapidly increased in complexity during the last few years, and combined multimodal therapy as well as multidisciplinary care with its inherent team decision-making is now considered standard [1]. The continuous and rapidly expanding range of potentially efficacious treatment options introduces therapeutic dilemmas about optimum management plans and how these should be presented to patients [2]. Today, there is a need to discuss the different diagnostic measures required to determine the exact stage and treatment options, which can include surgeons, radiotherapists, medical and clinical oncologists, histopathologists, nurse specialist and palliative care physicians [3].

Multidisciplinary team is defined as a collaborative approach to treatment planning, incorporating both clinical and supportive care input and considering all potential treatment options suitable for the individual patient [4].

The concept of MDT was formally introduced into UK practice during the 1990s. A major impetus was given by the publication of the Calman–Hine report in 1995 and the consequent drive to ensure that all patients with cancer, no matter where they might live, and to whom they might have been referred, would have equal access to a high and uniform standard of care [2].

The Calman–Hine report recommended major organisational changes, including more team working among those providing treatment and care, it was the first health policy to cover such a large and complex disease area, and it led to National service frameworks for other diseases [5].

It was followed by similar reviews in Scotland, Northern Ireland, and detailed report on cancer services in Wales. No reliable figures exist, but it is estimated that less than 20 % of all patients with cancer in England were managed in the context of

M. Innocenzi • G. D'Eramo (✉)
Department of Urology, University Sapienza, Viale Policlinico 155, 00161 Rome, Italy
e-mail: michele.innocenzi@uniroma1.it; giuseppe.deramo@uniroma1.it

V. Gentile et al. (eds.), *Multidisciplinary Management of Prostate Cancer*,
DOI 10.1007/978-3-319-04385-2_1, © Springer International Publishing Switzerland 2014

a specialist team a decade ago, and now over 80 % of such patients are managed in this way [6].

The seven principles of Calman–Hine report were:

- Access to uniform high-quality care in the community or hospital
- Early identification of cancer and availability of national screening programmes
- Patients to be given clear information at all stages
- Services to be patient centred
- Centrality of primary care and effective communications
- Psychosocial aspects of care are important
- Cancer registration and monitoring of treatment and outcome are essential

These principles mainly focused on the patients and their needs, placing them at the heart of the policy, in response to many accounts of unsatisfactory experiences from patients with cancer. The first principle has been quoted widely and remains an ambitious statement of the goals of this policy. The other principles covered important issues such as early identification of cancer, availability of national screening programmes, centrality of primary care, and monitoring of incidence, management, and outcomes through cancer registration [7].

The most radical and far-reaching feature of the policy was its challenge to the way many NHS clinical services had previously been organised. Calman–Hine required a fundamental shift from a substantially general service model, backed by specialist oncologists, into an overtly specialist cancer service [8].

The model proposed that all patients with cancer were seen by specialists in their cancer type. These specialists, surgeons or physicians, were required to work closely with colleagues in multidisciplinary teams composed of diagnostic disciplines, surgical and non-surgical oncologists, and nurse specialists. The intention was that team members, and the team as a whole, were to be specialists in the type of cancer concerned and to jointly decide on the management of individual patients. Thus, the policy sought a double transformation from patient access direct to specialists rather than generalists and from clinicians working individually (who choose whether to refer patients on to colleagues) to an overtly multidisciplinary model [9].

MDT work is widely accepted in many other countries, e.g. USA, Australia, and some countries in Europe, all of which have comparable initiatives to those listed above [10–12].

1.2   Multidisciplinary Team

The multidisciplinary team (MDT) is defined as a group of people of different healthcare disciplines, which meets together at a given time to discuss a given patient, each of them is able to contribute independently to the diagnostic and treatment decision about the patient. In general, surgeon, radiologist, and medical oncology dignify the core member of the team.

The National Breast Cancer Center has developed a set of five Principles of Multidisciplinary care providing a flexible approach to the implementation of MDC for patients with cancer. These principles emphasise the importance of standardised team approach, good communication, access to the full range of possible therapies, maintenance of standards of care and involvement of the patient in the decision-making process [13, 14].

Theoretically, MDT working should ensure an effective coordination, the best quality as well as a good continuity of patient care by bringing together key professionals with all necessary knowledge, skills, and experience. MDT working would thereby ensure high-quality diagnosis, evidence-based decisionmaking, optimum treatment planning, and delivery of care [15].

Specific participation is dependent on the type of tumour being discussed, the goals of the MDT as outlined earlier, and whether the meeting is to discuss diagnosis or treatment. One multidisciplinary discussion with all involved specialities is more effective and the joint decision more accurate than the sum of all individual opinion. A MDT is also an ideal learning opportunity for junior doctors and other professional figures. Patients are treated according to the same guidelines and the same standards regardless of which figure the patient was initially referred to. MDTs allow for the necessary investigation to be incorporated in the diagnostic process in order to prevent unnecessary or repented investigations to be performed [16].

A solution to reduce delays in diagnosis is the implementation of diagnostic assessment clinics. Such clinics provide a single point of access for the assessment of patient with suspected cancer, with access to diagnostic services and multidisciplinary consultation in a single location [17].

Gagliardi et al., in a systematic review of studies evaluating diagnostic assessment clinics, found that they reduce the time to diagnosis, which decreases patient anxiety and increases their satisfaction [18].

For a successful MDT care are needed team philosophy, leadership, dynamics, communication, and workload; of these criteria, good leadership is a prerequisite for effective team work, and MDTs need a leader to spur participation of team members [19]. Characteristics of a good leader include the ability to communicate well with team members and to use a participatory management leadership style, meaning that they should not only be able to get input from different members, utilising their input to reach group consensus and guide decisions, but also be able to make independent decisions when the situation arises. MDTs across several countries are most commonly led by surgeons; however, a system of rotating leadership of the team has been shown to reduce inter-professional conflicts and to improve team working and team morale within MDT. Overall team work is more successful when decision-making is visible and participative [20].

Factors that influence treatment decisions include disease stage, co-morbid health status, and patient preferences; in fact, the most common reason for an MDT decision being changed was where patients' co-morbid health status had not been sufficiently considered at the meeting [21].

In a study of 2005, Blazeby et al. show that 15.1 % of treatment decisions made at the upper gastrointestinal MDT meetings at United Bristol Healthcare Trust were not implemented (95 % confidence intervals 11.1 % to 20.0 %). Reasons for MDT decisions changing were mostly related to lack of information concerning patients' wishes or co-morbid disease and only eight decisions changed because unexpected metastatic disease was discovered at surgery. The author concluded that more information on co-morbidity and patient choice should be made available to MDTs to optimise decision-making [22].

The key point of each MDT is the presentation of cases; all relevant patient information should be presented in the most efficient and concise way. Presentation can be verbal, better if supported by a projection on a screen of the investigations until then performed. Professionals attending MDTs must ensure that their contribution remains relevant and concise [23].

The patient has to be involved in this decision-making process. However, if a single medicine presents the available options to the patient, there may be a relevant bias. It may be better for the different specialists to discuss the options with the patients in a combined clinic. In a study of Hack et al., the women with breast cancer that were actively involved in decision-making at diagnosis demonstrated an higher overall quality of life 3 years after diagnosis [24].

The recent institution of Virtual Multidisciplinary Teem (vMDT) has been introduced to resolve the economical and organisational problems of MDT. In fact, the improvement given to patient by MDT meetings, ensuring equality of access to high-quality care, is not without costs, both direct and indirect, and there is also evidence that some teams operate more effectively than others. One of the most reported problems in current practice is the need for member of team to meet regularly in order to discuss patients.

A vMDT meeting involves participants who may, or may not, be part of a permanent team and who interact with each other non-simultaneously using shared clinical data. They may operate at a local or National level and their remit is not necessarily confined to tumours presenting at a particular anatomical site [25].

1.3 The Impact of Mutlidisciplinary Team

Multidisciplinary team are assuming increasing importance in the delivery of cancer care. The goal of MDT is to review individual patients and to make recommendations about best management.

In 1996, the UK Department of Health published Improving Outcomes in breast cancer [26]; similar guidance for colorectal, lung, gynaecological, and upper gastrointestinal cancer followed [27–30].

Implementation of MDT has the potential to change treatment decision. In a study, Baldwin et al. reported an increase in the use of breast-conserving surgery for women who receive a preoperative multidisciplinary approach [31].

Forrest et al. compared two groups of patients with inoperable non-small cell lung cancer who were treated before (1997) and after (2001) introduction of MDT. In 2001, 23 % of patients received chemotherapy treatment compared with 7 % of patients in 1997. On follow-up, 116 of the 117 patients diagnosed in 1997 had died compared with 116 of 126 patients diagnosed in 2001. Median survival was significantly higher in patients treated in 2001 compared with those treated in 1997 (6.6 vs. 3.2 months) [32].

Katz et al., in a study of 2009 about a treatment of pancreatic adenocarcinoma, showed an increase of long-term survival of 329 patients who underwent surgical resection of their primary pancreatic adenocarcinoma. They attribute this result to the use of objective criteria for the selection of patients for surgery, a standardised approach to the technical aspects of the operation, an institutional emphasis on multimodality therapy, and the frequent use of neoadjuvant treatment sequencing [33].

Ganesan et al. between 2005 and 2006, about 400 patients with confirmed or suspected ovarian cancer, 108 cases were referred for discussion in the weekly clinico-pathology meeting for various indications. Ninety-one of the 108 cases discussed were available for analysis; 75.8 % of cases were initially diagnosed as epithelial ovarian cancers. In 48 of 91 cases (52 %), there was an alteration in the diagnosis as a direct result of discussion in the meeting; in 20 of 91 cases (22 %), the therapeutic indication were modified after MDT meeting [34].

Kee et al. in a study of 2004 valued MDT decision making. They reviewed 221 cases of lung tumour; in 39 % of cases, the initial treatment recommendation offered by the individual clinician before multidisciplinary team discussion was different from the final group decision. In 50 of these cases, the team discussion did not change the mind of the clinician about his or her preferred treatment. In 62 % of cases, the clinician subsequently concurred with the team choice of treatment [35].

Greer et al., in a study of 2010, reviewed in MDT 741 patients with gynaecological tumour. Of the 526 pathology reviews, 27 % had a change in diagnosis; this discrepancy altered clinical management 74 % of the time (20 % of all reviews). Of the 215 radiology presentations, 89 % were reviewed to confirm recurrent or persistent disease; malignant disease was confirmed 74 % of the time [36].

Gatcliff et al. in 2008 reviewed 153 patients. Alterations were made in 53 cases. Major alterations ($n = 13$) predominantly resulted from pathology reassignments. Minor alterations ($n = 40$) resulted from pathology, staging, radiology, and surgical team clarifications [37].

Chang et al. analysed 75 consecutive women with 77 breast lesions examined in consultation in a multidisciplinary breast cancer centre between January and June 1998 in Pennsylvania cancer centre. For the 75 patients, the multidisciplinary panel disagreed with the treatment recommendations from the outside physicians in 32 cases (43 %) and agreed in 41 cases (55 %). For the 32 patients with a disagreement, the treatment recommendations were breast-conservation treatment instead of mastectomy ($n = 13$; 41 %) or re-excision ($n = 2$; 6 %); further workup instead of immediate definitive treatment ($n = 10$; 31 %); treatment based on major change in diagnosis on pathology review ($n = 3$; 9 %); addition of post-mastectomy radiation treatment ($n = 3$; 9 %); or addition of hormonal therapy ($n = 1$; 3 %). MDT led to change treatment in 43 % of cases examined [38].

1.4   Medico-legal Implications of Group Decision

Western society is becoming more litigious, as indicated by increasing medico-legal claims over the last two decades across jurisdictions. Given these factors, medico-legal actions will inevitably be brought against decision made in MDT. However, the small number of malpractice litigation involving MDT suggests that they are a medico-legally safe decision-making process, and to the extent that team discussions have become the standard of care, clinicians remain obliged to continue managing their patients via this useful team [39].

The decisions made in MDT meetings are associated with an unconscious bias within the group, which despite best intentions can affect individual decisions as given below:

- Many participants will easily agree to a specific treatment option only when the benefit of that choice is obvious and much better than another option.
- The risk of an adverse event caused by a prescribed treatment affects individual medical decision-making more than does any probability of a benefit for the same patient.
- Single components of a diverse non-conformant treatment strategy are more useful in terms of outcome when considered as part of the entire strategy. This situation is relevant for multistep individualised strategies that are put forward for difficult clinical cases.

Given that this type of decision-making forum is quite a recent development, many participating doctors may be unaware of their medico-legal responsibilities. To succeed in a tort action in negligence, the patient must first prove that the doctor owed them a duty of care. This duty to take reasonable care arises from the professional patient–doctor relationship and is evident in the traditional face-to-face consultation [40]. Changes to the way doctors interact with patients, such as teleconferencing and email consultations, have widened the methods by which this relationship may be formed. The greatest danger is likely to occur in discussion-only clinics in which most doctors never meet the patients who are discussed. Despite this absence of personal contact, the doctors in the meeting still attract a legal duty to take reasonable care in exercising their judgement and will be potentially liable in the event that negligent advice results in injury or damage to a patient [41].

In Australia, patients are usually unaware that treatment management has been reviewed formally at scheduled MDT attended by health professionals with whom they have had no contact. Patients whose disease details have been de-identified do not necessarily need to be informed of MDT decisions [42].

Responsibility should be clearly identified for every person who is contributing to the multidisciplinary decision, with a common agreement that serves as a guideline for governing subsequent discussion about clinical interventions in complex cases [39] (Fig. 1.1).

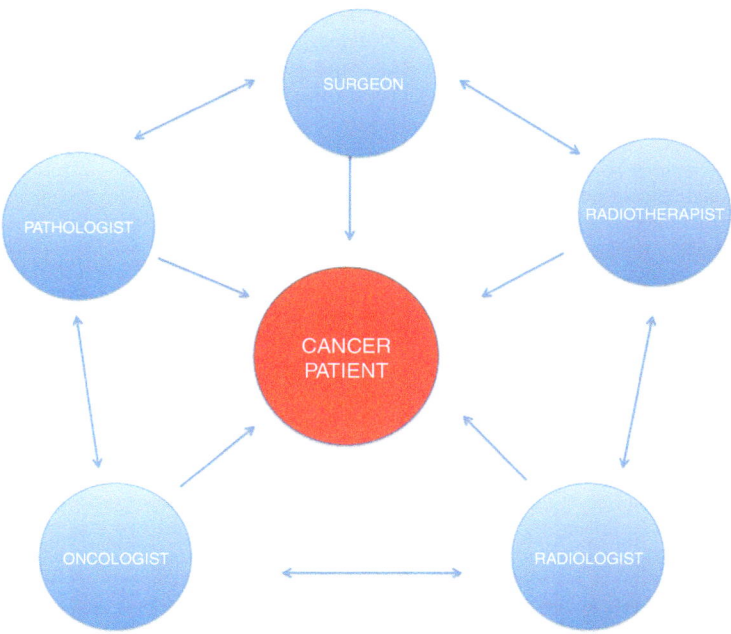

Fig. 1.1 An example of multidisciplinary team approach

References

1. Gouveia J, Voleman MP, Haward R et al (2008) Improving cancer control in the European Union: conclusions from the Lisbon round-table under the Portuguese EU presidency, 2007. Eur J Cancer 44:1457–1462
2. Haward RA (2003) Using service guidance to shape the delivery of cancer services: experience in the UK. Br J Cancer 89(suppl 1):S12–S14
3. Carter S, Garside P, Black A (2003) Multidisciplinary team working, clinical networks, and chambers; opportunities to work differently in the NHS. Qual Saf Health Care 12(suppl 1): i25–i28
4. Valdagni R, Salvioni R, Nicolai N et al (2005) In regard to Kagan: "The multidisciplinary clinic" (Int J Radiat Oncol Biol Phys 2005;61:967-968). Int J Radiat Oncol Biol Phys 63: 309–310
5. Department of Health (2004) Manual for cancer services 2004. Department of Health, London
6. Goolam-Hossen T, Metcalfe C, Cameron A et al (2011) Waiting times for cancer treatment: the impact of multi-disciplinary team meetings. Behav Inform Technol 30:467–471
7. Haward RA (2006) The Calman–Hine report: a personal retrospective on the UK's first comprehensive policy on cancer services. Lancet Oncol 7:336–346
8. Department of Health (2000) New cancer research co-ordinating centre, Leeds. Press Release, Department of Health, Nov 17, 2000
9. Halm EA, Lee C, Chassin MR (2002) Is volume related to outcome in health care? A systematic review and methodologic critique of the literature. Ann Intern Med 137:511–520
10. Ripathy D (2003) Multidisciplinary care for breast cancer: barriers and solutions. Breast J 9:60–63

11. Zorbas H, Barraclough B, Rainbird K et al (2003) Multidisciplinary care for women with early breast cancer in the Australian context: what does it mean? Med J Aust 179:528–531
12. Mission Interministerielle pour la Lutte contre le Cancer (2003) Cancer: a nation-wide mobilization plan (the French Cancer Plan). Mission Interministerielle pour la Lutte contre le Cancer, Paris (in French)
13. Scholnik AP, Arnold DJ, Gordon DC et al (1986) A new mechanism for physician participation in a tumor board. Prog Clin Biol Res 216:337–343
14. National Breast Cancer Centre (NBCC) (2003) Multidisciplinary care in Australia: a national demonstration project in breast cancer. NBCC, New South Wales, Australia
15. Lamb BW, Brown KF, Nagpal K et al (2011) Quality of care management decisions by multidisciplinary cancer teams: a systematic review. Ann Surg Oncol 18:2116–2125
16. Caplan GA, Williams AJ, Daly B et al (2004) A randomized, controlled trial of comprehensive geriatric assessment and multidisciplinary intervention after discharge of elderly patients in an emergency department- the DEED II study. J Am Geriatr Soc 52(9):1417–1423
17. Bydder S, Hasani A, Broderick C, Semmens J (2010) Lung cancer multidisciplinary team meetings: a survey of participants at a national conference. J Med Imag Radiat Oncol 54: 146–151
18. Gagliardi AR, Wright FC, Davis D (2008) Challenges in multidisciplinary cancer care among general surgeons in Canada. BMC Med Inform Decis Mak 8:59. doi:10.1186/1472-6947-8-59
19. Sidhom M, Poulsen M (2008) Group decisions in oncology: Doctors' perceptions of the legal responsibilities arising from multidisciplinary meetings. J Med Imag Radiat Oncol 52(3): 287–292
20. Haward R, Amir Z, Borrill C et al (2003) Breast cancer teams: the impact of constitution, new cancer workload, and methods of operation on their effectiveness. Br J Cancer 89(1):15–22
21. McCulloch P, Ward J, Tekkis PP (2003) Mortality and morbidity in gastro-oesphageal cancer surgery: initial results of ASCOT multicentre prospective cohort study. Br Med J 327:756–761
22. Blazeby JM, Wilson L, Metcalfe C et al (2006) Analysis of clinical decision-making in multidisciplinary cancer teams. Ann Oncol 17(3):457–460
23. Ruhstaller T, Roe H et al (2006) The multidisciplinary meeting: an indispensable aid to communication between different specialities. Eur J Cancer 42:2459–2462
24. Hack TF, Degner LF, Watson P et al (2006) Do patients benefit from participating in medical decision making? Longitudinal follow-up of women with breast cancer. Psychooncology 15:9–19
25. Munro AJ, Swartzman S (2013) What is a virtual multidisciplinary team (vMDT)? Br J Cancer 108(12):2433–2441
26. NHS Executive (1996) Improving outcomes in breast cancer: the manual. Department of Health, Leeds
27. NHS Executive (1997) Improving outcomes in colorectal cancer: the manual. Department of Health, Leeds
28. NHS Executive (1998) Improving outcomes in lung cancer: the manual. Department of Health, Leeds
29. NHS Executive (1999) Improving outcomes in gynaelogical cancer: the manual. Department of Health, Leeds
30. NHS Executive (2001) Improving outcomes in upper gastrointestinal cancer: the manual. Department of Health, Leeds
31. Baldwin LM, Taplin SH, Friedman H, Moe R (2004) Access to multidisciplinary cancer care: is it linked to the use of breast-conserving surgery with radiation for early-stage breast carcinoma? Cancer 100:701–709
32. Forrest LM, McMillan DC, McArdle CS, Dunlop DJ (2005) An evaluation of the impact of a multidisciplinary team, in a single centre, on treatment and survival in patients with inoperable non-small-cell lung cancer. Br J Cancer 93(9):977–978

33. Katz MH, Wang H, Fleming JB et al (2009) Long-term survival after multidisciplinary management of resected pancreatic adenocarcinoma. Ann Surg Oncol 16(4):836–847. doi:10.1245/s10434-008-0295-2
34. Ganesan P, Kumar L, Hariprasad R et al (2008) Improving care in ovarian cancer: the role of a clinico-pathological meeting. Natl Med J India 21(5):225–227
35. Kee F, Owen T, Leathem R (2004) Decision making in a multidisciplinary cancer team: does team discussion result in better quality decisions? Med Decis Mak 24:602–613
36. Greer HO, Frederick PJ, Falls NM et al (2010) Impact of a weekly multidisciplinary tumor board conference on the management of women with gynecologic malignancies. Int J Gynecol Cancer 20(8):1321–1325
37. Gatcliffe TA, Coleman RL (2008) Tumor board: more than treatment planning—a 1-year prospective survey. J Cancer Educ 23(4):235–237
38. Chang JH, Vines E, Bertsch H et al (2001) The impact of a multi-disciplinary breast cancer center on recommendations for patient management: the University of Pennsylvania experience. Cancer 91:1231–1237
39. Weiss N (2004) E-mail consultation: clinical, financial, legal, and ethical implications. Surg Neurol 61:455–459
40. Olick RS, Bergus GR (2003) Malpractice liability for informal consultations. Fam Med 35:476–481
41. Kuszler PC (1999) Telemedicine and integrated health care delivery: compounding malpractice liability. Am J Law Med 25:297–326
42. Dix A, Errington M, Nicholson K, Powe R (1996) Laws for the medical profession in Australia, 2nd edn. Butterworth-Heinemann, Melbourne

Prostate Cancer Units: How and Why

Stefano Salciccia, Alessandro Sciarra, and Valeria Panebianco

2.1 Bases for the Development of Prostate Cancer Units

Prostate cancer (PC) is established as one of the most important medical problems facing the male population. PC is the most common solid neoplasm (214 cases per 1,000 men) and the second most common cause of cancer death in men [1].

Its management involves several complex issues for both clinicians and patients. An early diagnosis is necessary to implement well-balanced therapeutic options and the correct evaluation can reduce the risk of overtreatment with its consequential adverse effects [2]. The optimal management for localized PC is controversial, with options including active surveillance, surgery, radiotherapy, and focal therapies. The management of the progressive disease after primary treatments and that of the advanced PC require a correct diagnostic evaluation and a therapeutic choice among radiotherapy, focal therapies, hormone therapies, chemotherapies, or other novel target treatments [3, 4].

Efficient organization of the national healthcare system can be a tool to help improve patient outcomes.

The natural history of PC from asymptomatic organ-confined disease to locally advanced, metastatic, and hormone-refractory disease describes the complexity of the biology of this tumor and justifies the need for a fluid collaboration between expert physicians.

S. Salciccia
Department of Gynecology, Obstetric and Urological Sciences, Policlinico Umberto I, University Sapienza Rome, Viale Del Policlinico 155, Rome 00161, Italy, Lazio
e-mail: stefi_sal77@tiscali.it

A. Sciarra
Department of Urology, University Sapienza, Viale Policlinico 155, Rome 00161, Italy

V. Panebianco (✉)
Department of Radiological Sciences, Oncology & Pathology, Sapienza University, Policlinico Umberto I, Viale Del Policlinico 155, Rome 00161, Italy, Lazio
e-mail: valeria.panebianco@uniroma1.it

V. Gentile et al. (eds.), *Multidisciplinary Management of Prostate Cancer*, DOI 10.1007/978-3-319-04385-2_2, © Springer International Publishing Switzerland 2014

Breast and Prostate cancer, respectively, are the most common cancers in women and in men, and different similarities have been underlined. The paradigm of the patient consulting a multidisciplinary medical team has been an established standard approach in treating breast cancer [5]. Such multidisciplinary approach can offer the same optional care for men with PC as it does for woman with breast cancer.

In other disease sites, multidisciplinary cancer clinics have been associated with decreased time from diagnosis to initiation of treatment, shorter time to completion of necessary pretreatment consultations, and fewer patient visits to clinicians' offices before initiation of care [6]. Multidisciplinary physician discussions have been shown to be associated with improved adherence to guidelines supported by the literature [7]. In a multidisciplinary prostate cancer clinic, newly diagnosed patients can simultaneously meet with urologic, radiation, and medical oncologists specializing in prostate cancer. Such a model of cancer care affords patients the opportunity to learn about all management options simultaneously and to discuss the recommendations of their treating physicians in an open and interactive fashion, allowing for shared decision making and a potential reduction in physician bias. Although it is important to note that such benefits have been demonstrated in oncological disease sites other than PC, in the last 10 years several experiences on multidisciplinary management of PC have been published showing several advantages in the management of PC: Valdagni et al. [8, 9], first in Italy (2004) to establish an MDT at Istituto Nazionale Tumori in Milano, recently reported their 6-years experience of an MDT prostate cancer clinic in Italy. Interestingly, they reported that most of the patients with PC were staged in the low-risk group and that number increased significantly from 40 % in 2006 to 61 % in 2009. Moreover, they reported a high percentage (about 80 %) of patients managed with active surveillance. This data is very interesting and it underlined that active surveillance, as reasonable approach today in patients with low-grade disease, is more often a therapeutic choice in an MDT where the methods are often standardized, for example, in the use of new biomarkers such as PCA3 (prostate cancer antigen 3) or pro-PSA or in the management of new imaging tools such as mMRI (multiparametric magnetic resonance). Similar results were reported by other authors from other countries such as the USA where the organization of the healthcare system could be different from Europe [10]. Aizer et al. reported their experience on 701 men with low-risk prostate cancer managed at three tertiary care centers in Boston [11]. In this study active surveillance in patients seen at a multidisciplinary clinic were double that of patients seen by individual practitioners (43 % vs. 22 %), whereas the proportion of men treated with prostatectomy or radiation decreased by approximately 30 % ($P < 0.001$). Interestingly, the number of physicians and specialties seen was significantly associated with the choice of active surveillance on univariate but not multivariate analysis. This data suggests that the multidisciplinary clinic itself, and not merely the number or type of physicians seen, is important to the shared decision-making process for selection of active surveillance and more generally to choose the best treatment for each individual patient. This aspect on MDT is very important because previous studies examining patterns of care in patients with low-risk PC have consistently shown that specialists prefer the modality of treatment that they themselves deliver [12, 13]. Physician bias in the management of prostate cancer was illustrated in a study in which urologists and radiation oncologists were asked as to how they would want to be treated if diagnosed with PC; 79 % of American urologists opted for radical prostatectomy and 92 % of American radiation oncologists chose radiation therapy. Similarly, in a survey of urologists and radiation oncologists in which several hypothetical PC scenarios were generated and questions regarding the recommended management were posed, both types of specialists commonly recommended the therapy that they were capable of offering and also tended to overestimate the benefit of definitive therapy [12, 13]. More interesting, the physician bias is also evident in the management of locally advanced disease in which patients undergoing surgery often require an adjuvant radiation therapy. Heather et al. in a survey of oncologists and urologists in the UK noted that the percentage of urologists who recommended surgery in this category of patients is relatively high (about 20 %) [14]. These data underlined the importance of physician bias when the patient with PC faces the specialist and the multidisciplinary approach can reduce drastically this bias as reported by Aizer's study on MDT [11].

Given that a multidisciplinary management can bring several advantages in the management of patients with PC, another important aspect is how the patient perceives a multidisciplinary management and which grade of satisfaction patients can have. Magnani et al. on 2012 reported a 6-years attendance of multidisciplinary prostate cancer clinics in Italy [8]. In their experience, to evaluate overall patient satisfaction, patients were periodically asked to complete a 10-item satisfaction questionnaire, covering several aspects of the patient's management including Physician Referral Service, waiting time, information given on health, and medical care. Patient satisfaction ratings were high: the investigators used a 7-point scale (in which a score of 1 designates "very poor quality," whereas a score of 7 indicates "very high quality"). Scores between 5 and 7 were achieved for all measured domains, including observance of privacy, care provided by technical/nursing staff, care provided by the clinical staff, information on health, and medical care provided. The management of PC is complicated by the multitude of management options, the lack of proven superiority of one modality of management, and the presence of physician bias. The available data suggest that implementation of multidisciplinary models of care for patients with cancer, when feasible, may be associated with high patient satisfaction rates and may alter practice patterns in ways that minimize physician bias [11].

2.2 How to Organize a Prostate Cancer Unit

Given that a multidisciplinary approach can bring many advantages in the management of patients with PC (Table 2.1), an important aspect is how to organize a Prostate Cancer Unit.

Table 2.1 Ten good reasons to support a Prostate Cancer Unit

1	PC is a very complex disease, involving diagnostic and therapeutic multidisciplinary decisions
2	Optimal and well-balanced information for PC cases requires a shift from a monodisciplinary to a synergic multidisciplinary approach
3	As Breast Cancer Units for breast cancer, multi-professional Prostate Cancer Units for PC are the best answer to manage patients and the complexity of their disease
4	Prostate Cancer Units offer the patient a complete, simultaneous, unambiguous, polispecialistic counseling on his disease, avoiding him to tour to different physicians
5	An MDT can provide a continuum of care for patients through early diagnosis, treatment planning in all stages of the disease, follow-up, prevention, and management of complications
6	Prostate Cancer Units connect a team whose members have specialist training in PC, spend relevant amount of time in working with PC, and have a high-level scientific qualification on PC
7	In Prostate Cancer Units the MDT can better propose the appropriate management options on the basis of the pathological reports, clinical and biochemical assessments, and the risk benefit evaluation
8	Prostate Cancer Units are in possession of or have easy direct access to all requirements for a complete, adequate, and high-level management of all phases of PC
9	Patients referred to a Prostate Cancer Unit receive more balanced information and decisions obtained in an open and interactive fashion, with all clinical specialists present at the same time
10	Patients referred to a Prostate Cancer Unit experience easier availability, enhanced coordination, and reduced delays to conclude the diagnostic and therapeutic item

Quality cancer care is complex and depends upon careful coordination between multiple treatments and providers and upon technical information exchange and regular communication flow between all those involved in treatment (including patients, specialist physicians, other specialty disciplines, primary care physicians, and support services) [15]. Traditional cancer treatment strategies began with individual consultations initiated by the internist or family practitioner with the relevant cancer specialist and subsequent patient referral to other specialists for specific cancer care treatments. An MDT comprises healthcare professionals from diverse disciplines whose goal of providing optimal patient care is achieved through coordination and communication with one another. Typically, MDT within oncology is disease focused, for example, head and neck, breast, thoracic, or genitourinary. The core disciplines integral to the multidisciplinary approach to cancer care are medical oncology, radiation oncology, surgical oncology, cancer site specialist, primary care, and nursing [16]. This type of structure ensures that the patient is informed and guided during and after treatment, from inpatient status to outpatient status, moving patient care prospectively. The benefits of a multidisciplinary approach to treating cancer may be particularly important in PC where there are so many treatment options available today including surgery, radiotherapy, hormonal therapy, focal therapy, or active surveillance and watchful waiting [17].

As suggested by Valdagni et al., a Prostate Cancer Unit is a place where men can be cared for by specialists in PC working together within a multi-professional team [18].

From October 2010 our hospital accepted the institution of a Prostate Cancer Unit. Our Prostate Unit was established in large size hospital, covering a population of more than 300,000 people.

The main aim of the unit was to provide a continuum of care for patients through early diagnosis, treatment planning in all stages of the disease, follow-up, prevention, and management of complications related to PC. Patients that can be followed by the Prostate Cancer Unit include cases in which the diagnosis is as yet unestablished but whose could benefit for an early diagnosis program; cases in which the diagnosis of PC is confirmed and whose can be considered for treatment planning; cases following primary treatment for discussion of further care; and cases in follow-up after or during treatment.

Following indications from previous experiences [18], we accepted some basic requirements for our Prostate Cancer Unit:

1. The unit is represented by a core team whose members have a specialist training in prostate disorders, spend a relevant amount of their time working with PC, undertake continuing professional education, and have a high-level scientific production on PC experimental and clinical research.

2. The core team include: two coordinators (one referred for the diagnostic and one for the clinical therapeutic management of PC) from any specialist of the team; urologists (spending 50 % or more of their working time in prostate disease, managing at least 100 PC cases per year, and carrying out at least 25 radical prostatectomies per year and at least one prostate clinic per week); urologist/radiologist dedicated to prostate biopsies (spending more than 70 % of his working time in prostate biopsies and performing more than 400 prostate biopsies per year); uropathologist (spending 30 % or more of his working time in prostate disease and analyzing at least 250 sets of prostate biopsies per year); radiation oncologists (spending 50 % or more of their working time in prostate disease and carrying out radiotherapy on at least 25 PC per year); medical oncologists (spending 30 % or more of their working time in prostate disease and managing at least 50 PC cases per year); and radiologists (with main experience in all aspects of prostate imaging, one using multiparametric magnetic resonance and ultrasonography and one as expert in nuclear medicine, and spending 50 % or more of his working time in prostate disease). Additional professional services also include a sexologist/andrologist, psychologist, palliative care specialist, and a clinical trials coordinator.

3. The Prostate Cancer Unit must be of sufficient size (number of specialists) to have more than 100 new diagnosed cases of PC coming under its care each year.

4. Research and scientific production is an important part of the activity of the Prostate Cancer Unit, such as also participation in clinical trials for the management of PC.

5. All specialists of the Prostate Cancer Unit core team organize and participate in multidisciplinary meetings every 10–14 days. Cases referred to the unit are discussed during the meeting. The MTD will propose the appropriate management options on the basis of pathological reports, clinical and biochemical

assessments, and risk benefit evaluations. The final decision will be made by patients informed by one of the clinicians.

6. The Prostate Cancer Unit is in possession of or has easy direct access to all requirements for a complete, adequate, and high-level management in all phases of PC.

The inclusion of radiologists in the core team of this unit is justified by the growing role of a morphologic-functional imaging (multiparametric magnetic resonance, PET-CT) for the management of PC. These two imaging tools have proven to be useful in the management of various aspects of PC natural history [19, 20].

A SEER-based study of more than 85,000 men with PC evidenced that in the general clinical practice the treatment decision had little relation to patient preferences but were predominantly associated with the specialty of the counseling clinician [21]. The primary advantage for patients referred to MTD organized into a Prostate Cancer Unit is to receive balanced information and decisions obtained in an open and interactive fashion, with all clinical specialists present at the same time. In the decision-making process for men with PC, this is one area in which the multidisciplinary approach can improve patient care.

The MTD approach guarantees a higher probability for the PC patient to receive adequate information on the disease and on all possible therapeutic strategies, balancing advantages and related side effects.

From the available evidences, patients with different cancers who are managed by MDT can experience better clinical outcomes [22, 23]. One of the first advantages described by patients referred to the Prostate Cancer Unit is an easier availability, enhanced coordination, and reduced delays to conclude the diagnostic and therapeutic item. This is likely to result in a better outcome for PC patients as early intervention is particularly crucial in cancer management [23].

The future of PC patients relies on a successful multidisciplinary collaboration between experienced physicians which can lead to important advantages in all the phases and aspects of PC management (Table 2.1).

The establishment of Prostate Cancer Units could provide financial saving, avoid inappropriate procedures, and improve outcomes delivering high-quality care to patients. These aspects are particularly relevant considering the high incidence of PC as one of the most important medical problems facing the male population.

References

1. Heidenreich A, Bellmunt J, Bolla M et al (2011) EAU guidelines on prostate cancer Part I. Eur Urol 59(1):61–71
2. Bellardita L, Donegani S, Spattezzi A, Valdagni R (2011) Multidisciplinary versus one-on-one setting: a qualitative study of clinicians' perceptions of their relationship with patients with prostate cancer. J Oncol Pract 7(1):1–5
3. Gomella L, Lin J, Hoffman-Censis J et al (2010) Enhancing prostate cancer care through the multidisciplinary clinic approach: a 15-year experience. J Oncol Pract 6(6):5–10

4. Van Belle S (2008) How to implement the multidisciplinary approach in prostate cancer management: the Belgian model. BJU Int 101(suppl 2):2–4
5. Montagut C, Albanell J, Bellmunt J (2008) Prostate cancer multidisciplinary approach: a key to success. Clin Rev Oncol Hematol 68S:32–36
6. Molyneux J (2001) Interprofessional teamworking: what makes teams work well? J Interprof Care 15:29–35
7. Borril C, West M, Shapiro D et al (2000) Team working and effectiveness in health care. Br J Health Care Manage 6:364–371
8. Magnani T, Valdagni R, Salvioni R, Villa S, Bellardita L, Donegani S, Nicolai N, Procopio G, Bedini N, Rancati T, Zaffaroni N (2012) The 6-year attendance of a multidisciplinary prostate cancer clinic in Italy: incidence of management changes. BJU Int 110(7):998–1003
9. Sommers BD, Beard CJ, D'Amico AV et al (2008) Predictors of patients preferences and treatment choices for localized prostate cancer. Cancer 113:2058–2067
10. Stewart SB, Bañez LL, Robertson CN, Freedland SJ, Polascik TJ, Xie D, Koontz BF, Vujaskovic Z, Lee WR, Armstrong AJ, Febbo PG, George DJ, Moul JW (2012) Utilization trends at a multidisciplinary prostate cancer clinic: initial 5-year experience from the Duke Prostate Center. J Urol 187(1):103–108
11. Aizer AA, Paly JJ, Zietman AL, Nguyen PL, Beard CJ, Rao SK, Kaplan ID, Niemierko A, Hirsch MS, Wu CL, Olumi AF, Michaelson MD, D'Amico AV, Efstathiou JA (2012) Multidisciplinary care and pursuit of active surveillance in low-risk prostate cancer. J Clin Oncol 30(25):3071–3076
12. Moore MJ, O'Sullivan B, Tannock IF (1988) How expert physicians would wish to be treated if they had genitourinary cancer. J Clin Oncol 6:1736–1745
13. Fowler FJ Jr, McNaughton Collins M, Albertsen PC, Zietman A, Elliott DB, Barry MJ (2000) Comparison of recommendations by urologists and radiation oncologists for treatment of clinically localized prostate cancer. JAMA 283(24):3217–3222
14. Payne HA, Gillatt DA (2007) Differences and commonalities in the management of locally advanced prostate cancer: results from a survey of oncologists and urologists in the UK. BJU Int 99(3):545–553
15. Fennell ML, Das IP, Clauser S, Petrelli N, Salner A (2010) The organization of multidisciplinary care teams: modeling internal and external influences on cancer care quality. J Natl Cancer Inst Monogr 2010(40):72–80
16. Basler JW, Jenkins C, Swanson G (2005) Multidisciplinary management of prostate malignancy. Curr Urol Rep 6(3):228–234
17. Wilt TJ, Ahmed HU (2013) Prostate cancer screening and the management of clinically localized disease. BMJ 346:f325
18. Valdagni R, Peter A, Bangma C et al (2011) The requirements of a specialist Prostate Cancer Unit: a discussion paper from the European School of Oncology. Eur J Cancer 47:1–7
19. Sciarra A, Barentsz J, Bjartell A, Eastham J, Hricak H, Panebianco V, Witjes JA (2011) Advances in magnetic resonance imaging: how they are changing the management of prostate cancer. Eur Urol 59(6):962–977
20. Picchio M, Giovannini E, Messa C (2011) The role of PET/computed tomography scan in the management of prostate cancer. Curr Opin Urol 21(3):230–236
21. Flessing A, Jenkins V, Cat S, Fallowfield L (2006) Multidisciplinary teams in cancer care: are they effective? Lancet Oncol 7(11):935–943
22. Houssami N, Sainsbury R (2006) Breast cancer: multidisciplinary care and clinical outcomes. Eur J Cancer 42(15):2480–2491
23. Davies AR, Deans DAC, Penman I et al (2006) The multidisciplinary team meeting improves staging accuracy and treatment selection for gastro-esophageal cancer. Dis Esophagus 19 (6):496–503

Comparison Between a Multidisciplinary and a Monodisciplinary Approach to Prostate Cancer: Our 1-Year Experience

3

Alessandro Sciarra, Vincenzo Gentile, and Alessandro Gentilucci

3.1 Introduction

Prostate cancer (PC) management involves several complex issues for both clinicians and patients. An early diagnosis is necessary to implement well-balanced therapeutic options and a correct evaluation can reduce the risk of overtreatment with its consequential adverse effects [1, 2]. The optimal management for localised PC is controversial, with options including active surveillance, surgery, radiotherapy and focal therapies. The management of the progressive disease after primary treatments and that of the advanced PC require a correct diagnostic evaluation and a therapeutic choice among radiotherapy, focal therapies, hormone therapies, chemotherapies or other novel target treatments [3].

Also, the natural history of PC, from asymptomatic organ-confined disease to locally advanced, metastatic and hormone-refractory disease, describes the complexity of the biology of this tumour and justifies the need for a fluid collaboration between expert physicians [4].

Breast and prostate cancer, respectively, are the most common cancers in women and in men, and different similarities have been underlined. The paradigm of the patient consulting a multidisciplinary medical team has been an established standard approach in treating breast cancer [5]. Such multidisciplinary approach can offer the same optional care for men with PC as it does for woman with breast cancer.

A. Sciarra (✉)
Department of Urology, University Sapienza, Viale Policlinico 155, 00161 Rome, Italy

Prostate Cancer Unit, Department Urology U Bracci, Policlinico Umberto I, University Sapienza of Rome, Viale Policlinico 155, 00161 Rome, Italy
e-mail: sciarra.md@libero.it

V. Gentile • A. Gentilucci
Department of Urology, University Sapienza, Viale Policlinico 155, 00161 Rome, Italy
e-mail: vincenzo.gentile@uniroma1.it; sciarra.md@libero.it

V. Gentile et al. (eds.), *Multidisciplinary Management of Prostate Cancer*,
DOI 10.1007/978-3-319-04385-2_3, © Springer International Publishing Switzerland 2014

A *multidisciplinary team* (MDT) comprises healthcare professionals from diverse disciplines whose goal of providing optimal patient care is achieved through coordination and communication with one another. A *Prostate Cancer Unit* is a place where men can be cared for by specialists in PC working together within a multiprofessional team [6].

3.2   Aim of the Analysis

The present study compares some results in terms of characteristics and distribution of PC cases, obtained by an MDT organised in a Prostate Cancer Unit, with those reported by a monodisciplinary urological unit, both operating in the same period and in the same Institution for the management of PC.

3.3   Characteristics of the Prostate Cancer Unit

From October 2010, our hospital officially accepted the institution of a Prostate Cancer Unit. Our Prostate Unit was established in a large size hospital, covering a population of more than 300,000 people.

The main aim of the Unit was to provide a continuum of care for patients through early diagnosis, treatment planning in all stages of the disease, follow-up, prevention and management of complications related to PC.

Patients who can be followed by the Prostate Cancer Unit include cases in which the diagnosis is as yet unestablished but whose could benefit from an *early diagnosis* programme (aged 40–70 years and with a prostate-specific antigen (PSA) serum levels >2.5 ng/ml); cases in which the diagnosis of PC is histologically confirmed and whose can be considered for *treatment planning*; cases following primary treatment for discussion of further care; and cases in *follow-up* after or during treatment.

Following indications from previous experiences [6], we accepted some basic requirements for our Prostate Cancer Unit:
1. The Unit is represented by a core team whose members have a specialist training in prostate disorders, spend a relevant amount of their time working with PC, undertake continuing professional education and have a high-level scientific production on PC experimental and clinical research.
2. The core team include two Coordinators (one referred for the diagnostic and one for the clinical therapeutic management of PC) from any specialist of the team; an urologist (spending 50 % or more of his working time in prostate disease, managing at least 100 PC cases per year and carrying out at least 30 radical prostatectomies per year and at least one prostate clinic per week); an urologist mainly dedicated in early diagnosis and prostate biopsies (spending more than 50 % of his working time in prostate biopsies and performing more than 400 prostate biopsies per year); an *uropathologist* (spending 30 % or more of his working time in prostate disease and analysing at least 250 sets of prostate

biopsies per year); *radiation oncologists* (spending 50 % or more of their working time in prostate disease and carrying out radiotherapy on at least 30 PC per year); *medical oncologists* (spending 30 % or more of their working time in prostate disease and managing at least 50 PC cases per year); and radiologists (with main experience in all aspects of prostate imaging, one using multiparametric magnetic resonance and ultrasonography and one as expert in nuclear medicine, and spending 50 % or more of their working time in prostate disease). Additional professional services also include a sexologist/andrologist, psychologist, palliative care specialist and a clinical trial coordinator.

3. The Prostate Cancer Unit must be of sufficient size (number of specialists) to have more than 100 diagnosed cases of PC coming under its care each year. The number of specialists could be increased in the following years.

4. Research and scientific production is an important part of the activity of the Prostate Cancer Unit, such as also participation into clinical trials for the management of PC.

5. All specialists of the Prostate Cancer Unit core team organise and participate to multidisciplinary meetings every 10–14 days. Cases referred to the Unit are discussed during the meeting. The MTD will propose the appropriate management options on the basis of pathological reports, clinical and biochemical assessments and risk–benefit evaluations. The final decision will be made by patients informed by one-two of the clinicians.

6. The Prostate Cancer Unit is in possession of or has easy direct access to all requirements for a complete, adequate and high-level management in all phases of PC.

The inclusion of radiologists in the core team of our Unit is justified by the growing role of a morphologic-functional imaging [multiparametric magnetic resonance (MRI), PET-computer tomography] for the management of PC.

The aim of our Prostate Cancer Unit was to offer balanced information and decisions for the patients, obtained in an open and interactive fashion, with all clinical specialists present at the same time.

3.4   Study Analysis

We analysed the characteristics of patients included in our Prostate Cancer Unit, some results obtained from the early diagnosis programme and the distribution of PC cases in the different treatment options, during the first year of institution of our Unit.

These data were compared with those obtained in a *monodisciplinary* urological service offered in the same period and in the same institution (Policlinico Umberto I Hospital, University Sapienza of Rome, Italy) to the patients. This urological service is organised in the Department of Urology of our institution. The same diagnostic and therapeutic tools were available for clinicians and patients considered in the Prostate Unit or in the monodisciplinary urological service. Patients referred to our institution are free to choose one of the two services.

3.5   Results

From January 2011 to April 2012, 292 cases with a mean age of 62.6 ± 11.0 years (median 64 years; range 43–76 years) were considered suitable and included by our MDT in the Prostate Cancer Unit (Group A). Of these, 145 were subjects in which the diagnosis was as yet unestablished, but whose could benefit from an early diagnosis programme and 147 were cases in which the diagnosis of PC was already histologically confirmed and whose could be considered for treatment planning or follow-up.

In the 147 cases with a previously established PC diagnosis, mean age was 67.6 ± 8.5 years (median 69 years, range 46–76 years) and the distribution on the basis of the *clinical staging* and *primary treatments* is reported in Table 3.1.

One hundred forty-five cases in which the diagnosis was unestablished (mean age 60.1 ± 7.6 years; median 57 years, range 43–69 years) were included in a early diagnosis programme for PC. Mean time for concluding all the initial programmes till the histological diagnosis at *prostate biopsy* (when indicated) was 22.3 ± 5.4 days (median 21 days, range 16–32 days). Clinical characteristics and diagnostic results of this population are presented in Table 3.2 and Fig. 3.1 and compared with those of a population (Group B) submitted, in the same period and institution, to a non-MDT organised monodisciplinary urological evaluation for the early diagnosis of PC. In Group B, mean time for concluding all the initial programmes till the *histological diagnosis* at prostate biopsy (when indicated) was 32.7 ± 6.6 days (median 33 days, range 23–42 days).

In both services (Prostate Cancer Unit = Group A and monodisciplinary urological evaluation = Group B), diagnostic tools available to determine whether to indicate a prostate biopsy were PSA serum determination, PCA3 determination, digital rectal examination (DRE) and *multiparametric MRI*. In both services, a 14-core random transrectal ultrasound-guided biopsy was used and also multiparametric MRI results could be used for additional targeted samples [7].

In particular, the rate of biopsy indications and that of PC positive biopsies was 64 % and 45 %, respectively, for cases included in Group A and 52 % and 41 % for cases included in Group B. Interviewing clinicians of the Prostate Cancer Unit and those of the monodisciplinary urological service, all cases indicated for biopsy in Group B should be considered for biopsy also in Group A, whereas only 76 % of cases indicated for biopsy in Group A should be confirmed in Group B.

Table 3.3 shows the characteristics of the newly diagnosed PC obtained in the two services (Groups A and B). The distribution of the newly diagnosed PC cases in risk categories [8] is shown in Fig. 3.2. A higher percentage of cases (47.6 %) referred to our MDT were in the low-risk group.

Figure 3.3 and Table 3.4 represent the distribution and the characteristics of 97 PC patients from Group A (42 newly diagnosed PC and 55 with a previously

Table 3.1 Characteristics of the 147 cases with a previously established PC diagnosis referred to our Prostate Cancer Unit

Parameter	Value
Age (years)	67.6 ± 8.5 (69), 46–76
Total PSA (ng/ml)	6.9 ± 23.2 (3.5), 0.003–146.0
Familiarity	24 (16.3)
Gleason score	
$\leq 7(3+4)$	115 (78)
$\geq 7(4+3)$	32 (22)
Staging	
Localised	95 (65)
Locally advanced	37 (25)
Metastatic	15 (10)
ADT-refractory	18 (12)
Therapies performed	
Radical prostatectomy (RP)	45 (30)
Radiotherapy (RT)	7 (5)
Hormone therapy (HT)	0 (0)
RP + RT	51 (35)
RP + HT	15 (10)
RT + HT	29 (20)

Values as number (% of cases) or Mean SD (median) and range
ADT androgen deprivation therapy

Table 3.2 Characteristics of cases with a unestablished diagnosis included in the early diagnosis programme of our Prostate Cancer Unit (Group A) compared with those of cases included in a similar programme of a monodisciplinary urological service (Group B)

Parameter	Group A	Group B
Number of cases	145	124
Age (years)	60.1 ± 7.6 (57), 43–69	65.4 ± 6.8 (63), 51–72
Familiarity	28 (19)	22 (18)
Total PSA (ng/ml)	10.8 ± 7.8 (6.7), 2.5–21.4	16.5 ± 8.4 (13.5), 4.7–28.5
Suspicious DRE	23 (16)	30 (24)
Number of multiparametric MRI	88 (61)	50 (40)
Indication for biopsy	93 (64)	64 (52)
Number of PCA3 test	25 (17)	14 (11)
Time to conclude the diagnostic item (days)	22.3 ± 5.40 (21), 16–32	32.7 ± 6.6 (33), 23–42

Values are reported as number (% of cases), mean SD (median) and range

established PC diagnosis enclosed for primary treatment planning) who were offered radical prostatectomy, radiotherapy or active surveillance as primary therapies. In particular, Fig. 3.3 shows that in the Prostate Cancer Unit (Group A), the indications for primary therapies were more distributed between *surgery* (51.5 %) and *radiotherapy* (45.4 %), also if the percentage of localised and locally advanced PC was different between the two treatment modalities. In all low-risk PC

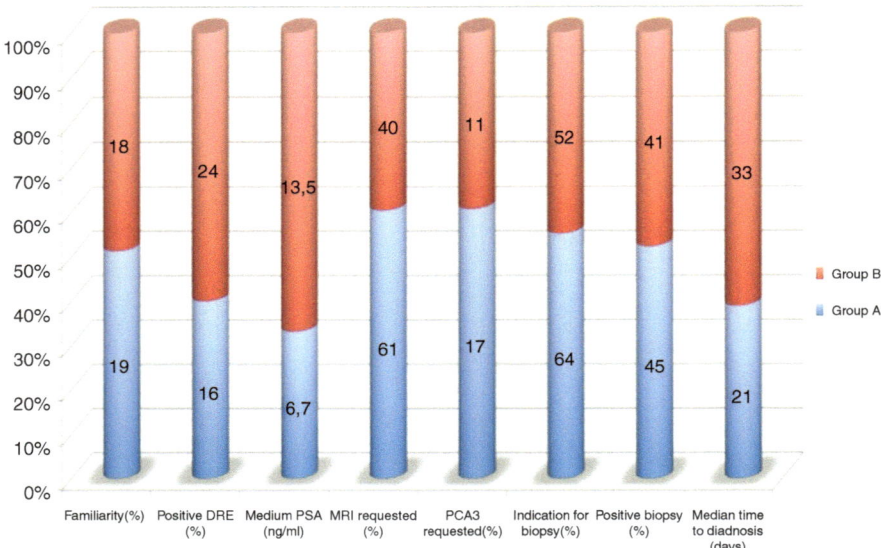

Fig. 3.1 Some characteristics of cases with an unestablished diagnosis of PC enclosed for an early diagnosis programme in Group A (Prostate cancer Unit) and Group B (monodisciplinary urological service)

Table 3.3 Characteristics of newly diagnosed PC obtained at biopsy from our Prostate Cancer Unit (Group A), compared to those obtained in a monodisciplinary urological service (Group B)

Parameter	Group A	Group B
Number of cases (%)	42 (45)	26 (41)
Age (years)	59.0 ± 5.3 (60), 48–68	64.2 ± 4.9 (63),53–72
Familiarity	9 (21)	4 (15)
Total PSA (ng/ml)	14.0 ± 6.6 (8.0), 2.8–21.4	17.2 ± 5.3 (14.0), 5.4–28.5
PCA3 positivity/number of tests	10/12 (83)	6/7 (86)
Suspicious DRE	11 (26)	8 (31)
Positive/number multiparametric MRI	41/42 (97)	10/10 (100)
Positivity at first biopsy	32 (76)	19 (73)
Positivity at re-biopsy	10 (24)	7 (27)
Gleason score		
≤7(3+4)	28 (67)	17 (64)
≥7(4+3)	14 (33)	9 (36)
Clinical staging		
Localised (T2N0M0)	31 (74)	17 (64)
Locally advanced (T3N0M0)	10 (24)	9 (36)
Metastatic (M+)	1 (2)	0 (0)

Values are reported as number (% of cases), mean SD (median) and range

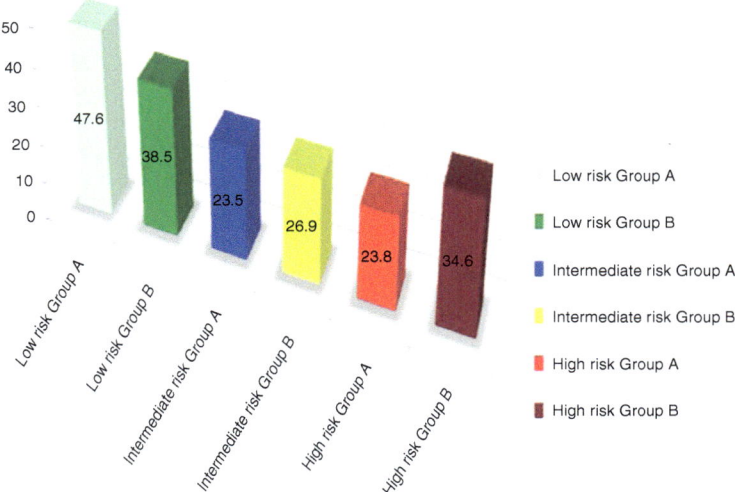

Fig. 3.2 Distribution of newly diagnosed PC in risk categories [8] (Group A = Prostate cancer Unit; Group B = monodisciplinary urological service)

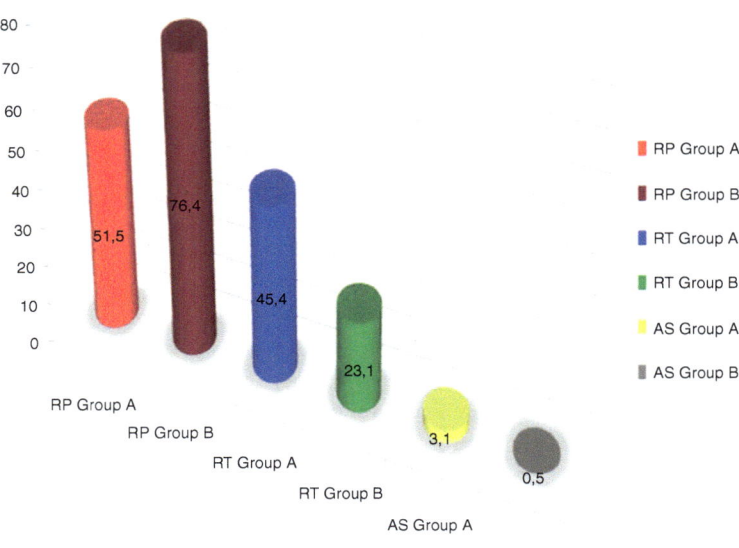

Fig. 3.3 Distribution of PC cases in the different indications for primary therapies (Group A = Prostate cancer Unit; Group B = monodisciplinary urological service)

Table 3.4 Ninety-seven cases (42 newly diagnosed PC and 55 with a previously established PC diagnosis enclosed for treatment planning) considered in Group A (Prostate Cancer Unit) for primary therapy [radical prostatectomy (RP), radiotherapy (RT) and active surveillance (AS)]

Parameter	RP in Group A	RT in Group A	AS in Group A
Number of cases (%)	50 (51.5)	44 (45.4)	3 (3.1)
Age (years)	61.4 ± 6.2 (60), 48–68	66.0 ± 5.8 (63), 52–70	56.0 ± 8.7 (52), 50–66
Total PSA (ng/ml)	11.4 ± 4.3 (8.5), 2.8–18.4	18.4 ± 6.3 (13.1), 8.5–20.0	2.7 ± 0.2 (2.8) 2.5–3.0
Gleason score			
$\leq 7(3+4)$	35 (70)	28 (64)	3 (100)
$\geq 7(4+3)$	15 (30)	16 (36)	0 (0)
Localised (T2N0M0)	38 (76)	19 (43)	3 (100)
Localised advanced (T3N0M0)	12 (24)	25 (57)	0 (0)

Characteristics of the PC cases distributed for different treatment options. Number (% of cases), mean SD (Median) and range

cases, *active surveillance* was offered as primary treatment; however, the percentage of cases who accepted was very low (3.1 %).

To evaluate patient satisfaction in the Prostate Cancer Unit, the cases were asked to complete a satisfaction questionnaire, covering: waiting time, accessibility and comfort to all procedures required, observance of scheduling, care by the clinical staff, information given by the staff and overall satisfaction. For each item, 5 ratings were possible [from 1 (very poor) to 5 (very high)]. At now, the mean scores ranged between 4.14 and 4.75 and the mean overall satisfaction score was 4.45.

3.6 Discussion

A SEER-based study of more than 85,000 men with PC evidenced that in the general clinical practice, the treatment decision has little relation to patient preferences but is predominantly associated with the speciality of the counselling clinician [9]. The primary advantage for patients referred to MTD organised into a Prostate Cancer Unit is to receive balanced information and decisions obtained in an open and interactive fashion, with all clinical specialists present at the same time. In the decision-making process for men with PC, this is one area in which the multidisciplinary approach can improve patient care.

The MTD approach guarantees a higher probability for the PC patient to receive an adequate information on the disease and on all possible therapeutic strategies, balancing advantages and related side effects.

From the available evidences, patients with different cancers who are managed by MDT could experience better clinical outcomes [10, 11]. One of the first advantages described by patients referred to the Prostate Cancer Unit is an easier availability, enhanced coordination and reduced delays to conclude the diagnostic and therapeutic item. This is likely to result in a better outcome for PC patients, as early intervention is particularly crucial in *PC management* [12].

However, a real significant advantage in terms of oncological results should be confirmed by long-term comparative analysis between an MDT and a monodisciplinary approach to the management of PC patients.

At now, only few studies in the literature described the results of a multidisciplinary prostate cancer clinic [13–15] and none of these compared results with those of a monodisciplinary team. Magnani et al. [13] reported a descriptive analysis of 6-year attendance of MDT Prostate Cancer Unit. As in our experience, a high percentage of low-risk cancers was associated to the early diagnosis programme, probably because of the anticipation of diagnosis. In our analysis, a higher rate of prostate biopsy indication when compared to that of the monodisciplinary team was found. Interviewing clinicians of the Prostate Cancer Unit (Group A) and those of the monodisciplinary urological service (Group B), all cases indicated for biopsy in Group B should be considered for biopsy also in Group A, whereas only 76 % of cases indicated for biopsy in Group A should be confirmed in Group B. Therefore, a more aggressive approach to the *diagnosis of prostate cancer* was shown in the Prostate Unit.

Regarding treatment planning, in particular, the very high percentage of cases who accepted an active surveillance (from 44 % in 2006 to 81 % in 2009) was reported by Magnani et al. [13]. Our experience shows a more balanced distribution of indications between surgery and radiotherapy when compared to the monodisciplinary team. In all low-risk cases, an active surveillance was proposed as a valid option; however, rate of *acceptability from patients* remained very low also in our Prostate cancer Unit.

References

1. Heidenreich A, Bellmunt J, Bolla M (2011) EAU guidelines on prostate cancer Part I. Eur Urol 59(1):61–71
2. Bellardita L, Donegani S, Spattezzi A, Valdagni R (2011) Multidisciplinary versus one-on-one setting: a qualitative study of clinicians' perceptions of their relationship with patients with prostate cancer. J Oncol Pract 7(1):1–5
3. Gomella L, Lin J, Hoffman-Censis J (2010) Enhancing prostate cancer care through the multidisciplinary clinic approach: a 15-year experience. J Oncol Pract 6(6):5–10
4. Van Belle S (2008) How to implement the multidisciplinary approach in prostate cancer management: the Belgian model. BJU Int 101(suppl 2):2–4
5. Montagut C, Albanell J, Bellmunt J (2008) Prostate cancer multidisciplinary approach: a key to success. Clin Rev Oncol Hematol 68S:32–36
6. Valdagni R, Peter A, Bangma C (2011) The requirements of a specialist Prostate Cancer Unit: a discussion paper from the European School of Oncology. Eur J Cancer 47:1–7
7. Sciarra A, Panebianco V, Ciccariello M (2010) Value of magnetic resonance spectroscopy imaging and dynamic contrast enhanced imaging for detecting prostate cancer foci in men with prior negative biopsy. Clin Cancer Res 16(6):1875.83
8. Heidenreich A, Bolla M, Joniau S (2012) Prostate cancer. In: European Association Urology guidelines. EAU, Arnhem, pp 9–10

9. Sommers BD, Beard CJ, D'Amico AV (2008) Predictors of patients preferences and treatment choices for localized prostate cancer. Cancer 113:2058–2067
10. Flessing A, Jenkins V, Cat S, Fallowfield L (2006) Multidisciplinary teams in cancer care: are they effective? Lancet Oncol 7(11):935–943
11. Houssami N, Sainsbury R (2006) Breast cancer: multidisciplinary care and clinical outcomes. Eur J Cancer 42(15):2480–2491
12. Davies AR, Deans DAC, Penman I (2006) The multidisciplinary team meeting improves staging accuracy and treatment selection for gastro-esophageal cancer. Dis Esophagus 19(6): 496–503
13. Magnani T, Valdagni R, Salvioni R (2012) The 6-year attendance of a multidisciplinary prostate cancer clinic in Italy: incidence of management changes. Br J Urol Int 110(7): 998–1003
14. Valdagni R (2011) Prostate cancer units: has the time come to discuss this thorny issue and promote their establishment in Europe? Eur Urol 60:1193–1196
15. Denis L (2011) Prostate Cancer Units: the patients' perspective. Eur Urol 60:1200–1201

Role of Pathology in the Multidisciplinary Management of Patients with Prostate Cancer

4

Rodolfo Montironi, Roberta Mazzucchelli, Marina Scarpelli, Antonio Lopez-Beltran, Andrea B. Galosi, and Liang Cheng

4.1 Introduction

A problem when handling and reporting radical prostatectomy specimens (RPS) is that cancer is often not visible at gross examination and the tumour extent is always underestimated by the naked eye. The challenge is increased further by the fact that prostate cancer is a notoriously multifocal and heterogeneous tumour. For the pathologist, the safest method to avoid undersampling of cancer is evidently that the entire prostate is submitted. Even though whole mounts of sections from RPS appear not to be superior to sections from standard blocks in detecting adverse pathological features, their use has the great advantage of displaying the architecture of the prostate and the identification and location of tumour nodules more clearly, with particular reference to the index tumour; further, it is easier to compare the pathological findings with those obtained from digital rectal examination (DRE), transrectal ultrasound (TRUS) and prostate biopsies [1–4].

The Ancona approach to the evaluation of the radical prostatectomies with special reference to the sampling and reporting of the prostate base/bladder neck and seminal vesicles.

R. Montironi (✉) • R. Mazzucchelli • M. Scarpelli
Section of Pathological Anatomy, Polytechnic University of the Marche Region, School of Medicine, United Hospitals, Via Conca 71, 60126 Torrette, Ancona, Italy
e-mail: r.montironi@univpm.it

A. Lopez-Beltran
Department of Surgery, Cordoba University Medical School, Cordoba, Spain

A.B. Galosi
Division of Urology, "Murri" General Hospital, Fermo, ASUR Marche, Italy

L. Cheng
Department of Pathology and Laboratory Medicine, Indiana University School of Medicine, Indianapolis, IN, USA

V. Gentile et al. (eds.), *Multidisciplinary Management of Prostate Cancer*,
DOI 10.1007/978-3-319-04385-2_4, © Springer International Publishing Switzerland 2014

This chapter is based on the Ancona (Italy) protocol for the evaluation of the RPS with complete sampling with whole mount sections. The protocol is the result of a close collaboration with the Universities of Cordoba (Spain) and Indiana (Indiana, IN, USA) and the implementation of the Ancona protocol gives clinical significance to our work of uropathologists, especially in the setting of a multidisciplinary management of patients with prostate cancer and of personalized medicine [2, 5].

Special reference is made here to the International Society of Urological Pathology (ISUP) Consensus Conference on Handling and Staging of Radical Prostatectomy Specimens [3]. Some of the authors of this chapter (R. Montironi, A. Lopez-Beltran and L. Cheng) greatly contributed to this conference, including in a role of co-organizers. The results of this conference reflects and to some extent incorporates the Ancona approach, and vice versa.

4.2   2009 International Society of Urological Pathology Survey and Consensus Conference

In order to identify the methods most commonly employed by urological pathologists worldwide, a Web-based survey on handling and reporting of radical prostatectomy specimens was distributed to 255 members of the International Society of Urological Pathology (ISUP). The ISUP survey was followed up with a consensus conference held in conjunction with the 2009 Annual Scientific Meeting of the United States and Canadian Academy of Pathology held in Boston, Massachusetts (Table 4.1) [3, 6–9]. The aim was to obtain consensus relating to the handling and reporting of radical prostatectomy specimens. Those who completed the electronic survey were invited to attend the consensus conference, which was held on 8 March 2009 [3].

Many recommendations of this consensus conference have already been incorporated into international guidelines, including the recent College of American Pathologists protocol and checklist for reporting adenocarcinoma of the prostate and the structured reporting protocol for prostatic carcinoma from the Royal College of Pathologists of Australasia [10, 11].

In response to the question relating to how much of the prostate should be blocked, >60 % of conference participants supported complete embedding, whereas >60 % also supported partial embedding. This apparent contradiction arose as several respondents selected both options depending on the situation. In view of this, it was concluded that both methods were considered acceptable. Pathologists have to balance the extra expense and time involved in processing entire specimens against the risk of missing important prognostic parameters and decide whether partial or complete embedding should be performed. There was consensus that if partial embedding is performed, a specific protocol should be followed and the methodology should be documented in the pathology report [3].

From the survey, a majority of respondents reported using standard blocks and only 16 % reported the use of whole mounts, for at least some slices. A minority

Table 4.1 Working groups (WG). International Society of Urological Pathology on handling and reporting of RP specimens

1. WG1, Handling of Radical Prostatectomy Specimens. R Montironi (Chair), H Samaratunga, L True
2. WG2, pT2 substaging and tumour volume in prostatectomy specimens. T Van der Kwast (Chair), M Amin, A Billis
3. WG3, Extraprostatic extension, lymphovascular invasion and locally advanced disease. PA Humphrey (Chair), C Magi-Galluzzi, AJ Evans
4. WG4, Seminal Vesicle and lymph node sampling. D Berney (Chair), T Wheeler, D Grignon
5. WG5, Surgical margins in radical prostatectomy specimens. J Epstein (Chair), L Cheng, P Hoon Tan

reported using both methods. On discussion at the consensus conference, it was considered that both standard blocks and whole mounts were acceptable for examination of radical prostatectomy specimens, although no ballot was taken on this point [3].

4.3   Total Versus Partial Embedding

For the pathologist, the safest method to avoid undersampling of cancer is evidently that the entire prostate is submitted. In some institutions, partial sampling is practiced. This requires that the pathologist adheres to a strict protocol, which may be somewhat cumbersome.

In 1994, a report on how prostate specimens were examined by American pathologists showed that only 12 % of pathologists embedded the entire prostate [12]. Since then the proportion of laboratories that use partial embedding has decreased. In a recent ENUP survey among 217 European pathologists from 15 countries, only 10.8 % used partial embedding routinely [13]. In some European countries, total embedding is even mandatory, according to national guidelines.

The recent study by Dr. Vainer et al. [14] analyses 238 RPS to determine whether significant prognostic information is lost when a partial sampling approach with standard cassettes is adopted, compared with total embedding. In their study, upon arriving at the pathology department, the prostate is partly divided by a cut in the mid-sagittal plane through the anterior surface, separating the two lobes for optimal fixation. The gland is then fixed for an additional 20 h in formic acid and 24 h in 4 % buffered formalin. The gross examination includes measurement in three dimensions, weighing the prostate after removal of the seminal vesicles, and separating the left from the right lobe after inking the anterior and the posterior halves with two different colours. Apical and basal slices of 5–10 mm, depending on the total size of the RPS, are cut horizontally, subsequently sliced parasagittally, and placed in cassettes with often more than one section per cassette. The remaining part of the prostate is cut horizontally in approximately 3-mm thick slices and placed in standard cassettes, ensuring laterality. Large slices are divided to fit standard cassettes. Finally, sections from the seminal vesicles (as a minimum the apex and a cross-section) are embedded. Post-fixation in 4 % formalin and embedding in paraffin are followed by 4-μm sectioning and staining with haematoxylin and eosin (number of cassettes/total slides: 18 to 76). For the purpose of the study, glass slides from every second horizontal slice are withheld (number of slides initially removed: 3 to 26, i.e. 29.9 %). The remaining slides are evaluated microscopically.

According to this group of researchers, such an approach decreases the laboratory workload by 30 %, and at the same time little information is lost with this procedure, overlooking features significant for the postoperative treatment in only 1.2 %. They conclude that partial embedding is acceptable for valid histopathological assessment.

The findings reported by Dr. Vainer et al. [14] are slightly better than those reported by others. Hall et al. [1] showed that by submitting only gross stage B cancer along with standard sections of the proximal and distal margins, the base of seminal vesicles and the most apical section (next to distal margin), 96 % of positive surgical margins and 91 % of instances of extraprostatic extension were detected, as compared with identification by complete microscopic examination. In the study by Cohen et al. [15] involving patients with clinical stage B carcinoma, each gland was serially sectioned with sections mounted whole on oversized glass slides. Using only alternate sections, there was a 15 % false-negative rate for extraprostatic extension. In a study by Sehdev et al. [4], cT1c tumours with one or more adverse pathological findings, such as Gleason score 7 or more, positive margins and extraprostatic extension, were compared using ten different sampling techniques. The optimal method consisted of embedding every posterior section and one mid-anterior section from the right and left sides of the gland. If either of the anterior sections had sizable tumour, all anterior slices were blocked in a second step. This method detected 98 % of tumours with Gleason score 7 or more, 100 % of positive margins and 96 % of cases with extraprostatic extension, through examination of a mean number of 27 slides. It was also shown that sampling of sections ipsilateral to a previously positive needle biopsy detected 92 % of Gleason score 7 or greater cancers, 93 % of positive margins and 85 % instances of extraprostatic extension, from a mean number of 17 slides.

4.4   The Ancona (Italy) Approach to the Evaluation of the Radical Prostatectomies

In the last few years, 3,000 RPS have been totally embedded and examined with the whole mount technique at the Section of Pathological Anatomy of the Polytechnic University of the Marche Region and United Hospitals, Ancona, Italy (Fig. 4.1) [2, 5].

The prostate is received fresh from the operating room. Its weight without the seminal vesicles and all three dimensions [apical to basal (vertical), left to right (transverse) and anterior to posterior (sagittal)] are recorded, the latter used for prostate volume calculation. To enhance fixation, 20 ml 4 % buffered formalin is

Fig. 4.1 Prostate gland and seminal vesicles examined with the whole mount technique

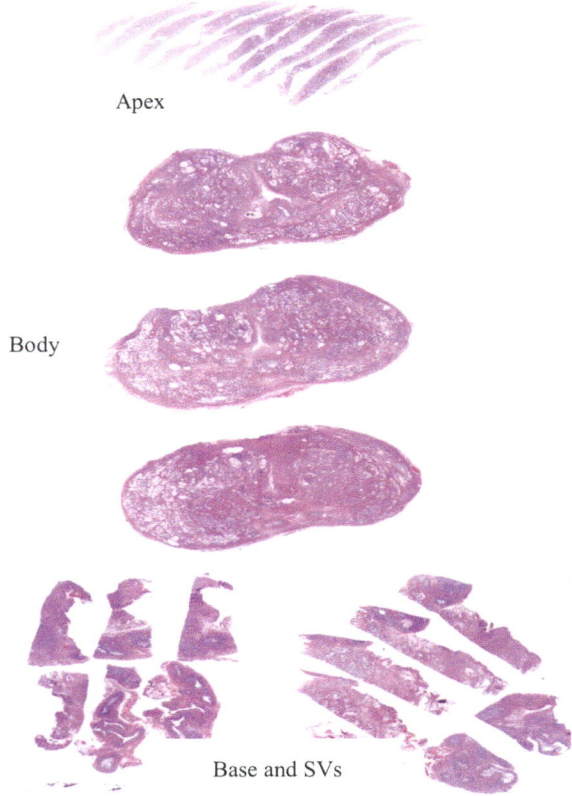

Apex

Body

Base and SVs

introduced into the prostate at multiple sites using a 23-G needle. To ensure homogenous fixation, the needle is inserted deeply and the solution injected while the needle is retracted slowly. The specimen is then covered with India ink and fixed for 24 h in 4 % neutral buffered formalin. After fixation, the apex and base (3-mm thick slices) are removed from each specimen and examined by the cone method. The prostate body is step-sectioned at 3-mm intervals perpendicular to the long axis (apical–basal) of the gland. For orientation, a cut with a surgical blade is made in the right part of each prostate slice. The seminal vesicles are cut into two halves (sandwich method) and processed in toto. The cut specimens are post-fixed for an additional 24 h in 4 % neutral buffered formalin and then dehydrated in graded alcohols, cleared in xylene, embedded in paraffin (the material is processed together with regular cassettes), and examined histologically as 5-μm thick whole mount haematoxylin and eosin (H&E) stained sections [2, 5].

The body of each prostate is represented with 3–6 whole mount slides, whereas the apex, base and seminal vesicles with 6–8 regular slides, totalling between 9 and 14 slides (In Dr. Vainer et al.'s study [14], up to 76 regular slides are needed to

Table 4.2 Comparison between Ancona experience and Dr. Vainer et al.'s study

Features	Ancona experience	Dr. Vainer et al.'s study
Prostate weight and size (and volume)	Yes (yes)	Yes (not mentioned)
Fixation enhancement	Formalin injection	Separating the two lobes
Inking of the surface	One colour; orientation with a cut on the right	Two colours, anterior and posterior halves
Pre-sectioning fixation (time)	4% Buffered formalin (24 h)	Acid formic (20 h) and 4 % buffered formalin (24 h)
Sectioning interval	3 mm (Apex and base: 3 mm)	Approximately 3 mm (Apex and base: 5–10 mm)
Sub-division of the slices of the prostate body	No (Whole mounts)	Yes, to fit standard cassettes
Seminal vesicles	Sandwich method (all included)	As a minimum the apex and a cross-section
Post-sectioning fixation (time)	4 % Buffered formalin (24 h)	4 % buffered formalin (not mentioned)
No. of cassettes/total slides (% examined)	9–14 (100 %)	18–76 (70 %)
Processing	As for regular size cassettes	Not mentioned
Slide size (section thickness)	7.5 cm by 5.0 cm (5 μm)	7.5 cm by 2.5 cm (4 μm)
Slide staining procedure	Manual	Not mentioned

examine the whole prostate). The time needed to section each specimen with an ordinary delicatessen meat slicer is 15–20 min. The time taken by a technician to cut all the blocks of an individual case is 30–40 min. The time needed by the pathologist to report a case ranges from 40 to 60 min. Since the slides do not fit into the current staining machines, the slides are manually stained. The paraffin blocks and glass slides are stored in dedicated containers because of their large size. The comparison between Dr. Vainer et al.'s and our approach is presented in Table 4.2 [14].

Slides with substandard sections, however with cancer still evaluable, were observed in 7 cases (0.23 % of RPS). Only in one case (0.03 %), the quality was so poor that the features could not be evaluated. An individual block had to be serially sectioned to visualize the entire inked surface in 15 cases (0.5 %). Immunohistochemistry (mainly the basal cell marker p63, racemase and Chromogranin A) was done, always successfully, in 30 cases (1 %), cutting from the whole mount section the part to be evaluated in 28, and using the whole mount section in the remaining two. A procedure was developed to search for residual cancer prostate cancer on pT0 radical prostatectomy after positive biopsy [16, 17]. When applied to 10 cases, a minute focus of cancer was successfully found in 8 [16].

The complete set of slides of each case is examined macroscopically and then microscopically and information on morphological items with diagnostic and prognostic importance is gathered (Figs. 4.2, 4.3, and 4.4) (Table 4.3) and

Fig. 4.2 Whole mount
section with a pT2a prostate
cancer (*Circled*)

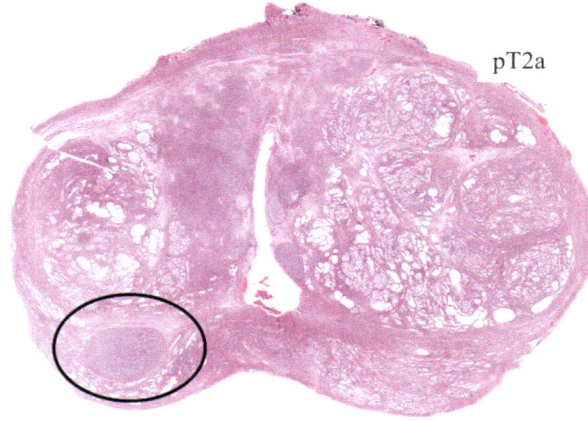

Fig. 4.3 Whole mount
section with a pT3a
(extraprostatic extension)
prostate cancer (*Arrow*)

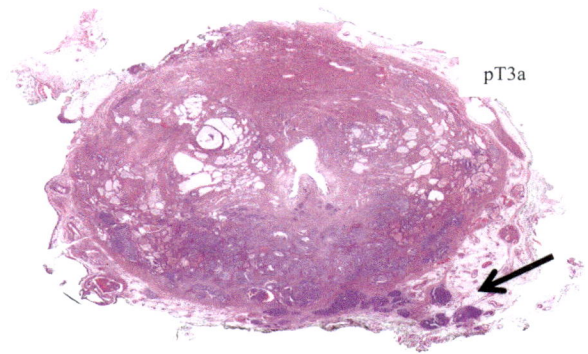

Fig. 4.4 Whole mount
section with a pT4 prostate
cancer invading the rectal
wall (*Arrow*)

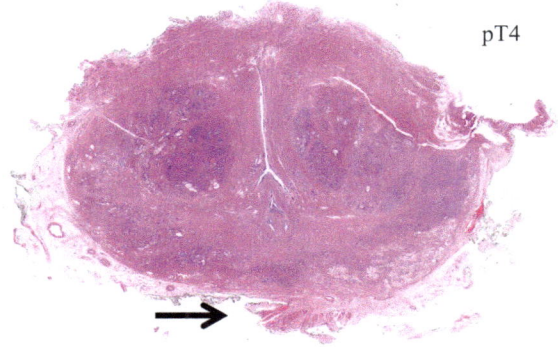

Table 4.3 Items evaluated when reporting radical prostatectomy specimens

1. Tumour multifocality (*Dominant or index tumor*)
2. Histological type
3. Grading according to the Gleason system (Original *vs. 2005 ISUP vs.* 2010 revision)
4. TNM stage, including surgical margin (SM) status (R) and LVI
5. Tumour volume

Table 4.4 Advantages with the Ancona (Italy) approach to the evaluation of the radical prostatectomies

1. Quality indicators of the surgical procedure: specimen integrity, including missing parts, capsular incision into tumour and benign glands at the surgical margins
2. Type of surgical procedure applied, i.e. nerve sparing; and previous surgical procedure, such as transurethral resection of the prostate
3. Presence of tissues other than prostate, i.e. rectal wall
4. Morphologic prognostic and predictive features, such as Gleason score, stage, surgical margin status and tumour volume
5. Comparison of pathological findings with digital rectal examination, transrectal ultrasound and prostate biopsies findings

interpreted in conjunction with clinical information and the macroscopic description of the specimen (Table 4.4).

Even though whole mounts of sections from RPS appear not to be superior to sections from standard blocks in detecting adverse pathological features [15], their use has the great advantage of displaying the architecture of the prostate and the identification and location of tumour nodules more clearly, with particular reference to the index tumour; further, it is easier to compare the pathological findings with those obtained from DRE, TRUS and prostate biopsies.

4.5 Combined Handling of Prostate Base/Bladder Neck and Seminal Vesicles in Radical Prostatectomy Specimens: *Our Approach with the Whole Mount Technique*

Following the 2009 ISUP consensus conference, our group has worked on issues related to handling and reporting of RPSs at the Section of Pathological Anatomy of the Polytechnic University of the Marche Region, Ancona, Italy, where a complete sampling procedure with coronal serial sectioning from the apex through the body to the base coupled with the whole mount technique is routinely applied. This procedure has given us important pieces of information related to the definition of insignificant vs. significant prostate cancer as well as to contemporary approaches in prostate cancer treatment, including active surveillance and focal therapy [5, 18, 19].

In the last 2 years, one of our main goals has been to further refine the analysis method of the prostate base/bladder neck, seminal vesicles and their junction with the prostate [20]. The reason has been the need for a more accurate and detailed histological evaluation of the whole area, which includes both the prostate base/bladder neck and seminal vesicles. The background has been that one of our group was probably among the first who defined histologically the prostate base and the bladder neck in a radical prostatectomy specimen at the World Health Organization co-sponsored International Consultation held in 1999 in Paris, France [21]. Its definition was based on the presence or absence of the prostate glands and the morphology of the smooth muscle bundles: prostate base when normal prostate glands are present, whereas bladder neck when such glands are absent and the smooth muscle bundles are coarse. This approach is now the foundation for the definition of the microscopic invasion of the bladder neck, which is considered as pT3a in the current 2009 TNM revision.

After examining several hundreds of RPSs, we have observed that the external boundaries, the shape and size of the prostate base/bladder neck area are related to the dimensions of the prostate gland and the relationship of the bladder wall with the prostate gland, and can vary from specimen to specimen. For instance, in some the basal surface can be slightly excavated or depressed while in others bulging and occasionally with a third lobe. Such anatomical variability also involves and influences the location of junction of the seminal vesicles with the prostate [20].

We have always discarded and therefore never adopted the shave approach because, when cancer is present, the relationship with the inked surface is not seen, thus reporting as positive surgical margin also situations in which the tumour does not actually touch the inked surface. We have to add a further reason for discarding this approach: a clear distinction between prostate base *vs.* bladder neck involvement, as defined above, is very difficult to achieve and therefore separation between a pT2 and pT3a cancer is impossible in certain situations [20].

For many years, we applied the cone approach (with sagittal sectioning) to a basal 3-mm thick slice. Typically, the diameter of the basal slice, whose shape was that of a disc or an ellipsoid, was approximately 3 cm in greatest diameter, i.e. such that its sagittal sections could be fit into a regular tissue cassette (dimensions: $30 \times 25 \times 4$ mm), but lower than the actual dimensions of the basal area whose size corresponds to the left to right (transverse) and anterior to posterior (sagittal) diameters of the gland. This approach allowed for the distinction of the prostate base from the bladder neck, but not for the examination of the whole basal surface. Another disadvantage with this approach was that, after removing the seminal vesicles, some prostate tissue containing the posterior part of the basal prostate remained buried in the most basal or proximal slice of the prostate body and therefore not examined histologically. This part usually contains the junction of the seminal vesicles with the prostate and also what some authors consider an intraprostatic component of the seminal vesicles [6]. This means that the cancer in this location might show adverse prognostic features that are not available for evaluation.

To avoid that the full spectrum of the morphologic features were not evaluable, we experimented an approach in which the RPSs were processed with complete sagittal sectioning from the right lateral aspect or margin of the specimen to the left margin, the slices still being cut at 3-mm interval. This approach allowed the simultaneous representation of the specimen from the apex to the tip of the seminal vesicles in the same whole mount sections [20]. However, this is possible for specimens whose length from the apex to the tip of the seminal vesicle is up to 6.3 cm, i.e. the maximum length of a large tissue cassette or megacassette (dimensions: $63 \times 47 \times 11$ mm). The disadvantage of the method is that the posterolateral aspects of the body of the prostate, i.e. a frequent location of prostate cancer, are not properly sampled and therefore evaluable for adverse prognostic features, including extraprostatic extension, and for the type of surgery operation done by the urologists, such as a nerve sparing procedure.

As a further step in our quest to accurately sample the region, we have evaluated and now adopted in the routine the following approach when the gland is fully fixed for at least 48 h, fixation being enhanced with formalin injection into the fresh specimen:

- The seminal vesicles, removed 1-to-2 mm away from the junction with the prostate, are sliced into two halves (sandwich method) and processed in toto together with the vas deferens in a single megacassette, or two depending on their size, and cut with the whole mount technique. The right seminal vesicle is identified with a cut made with a surgical blade.
- An approximately 1.5-cm thick slice comprising the entire base/bladder neck region comprising the 1-to-2 mm stump of seminal vesicles is removed from the body of the prostate. This part is then examined with sagittal sectioning at a 3-mm interval. The sagittal slices are then processed with the whole mount technique in two megacassettes, one for the right part and the other for the left part. The sagittal slice obtained from the basal slice and the seminal vesicle are sampled together when the specimen can be processed in a single megacassette (Figs. 4.5 and 4.6).
- The body of the prostate and the apex are still processed as previously reported.
- The body of each prostate, the base/neck area, and seminal vesicles are represented with 6–8 whole mount slides, whereas the apex with 2–4 regular slides, totalling between 8 and 12 slides (In a Dr. Vainer et al.'s study [14], up to 76 regular slides are needed to examine the whole prostate).
- When needed, immunohistochemistry has been successfully applied.

We have used this approach in more than 100 RPSs [20]. So far, we have seen neither disadvantages nor drawbacks. Its implementation does not require an additional amount of work from the technicians' side. When the findings are compared with the previous handling approach, several advantages have been fully appreciated in terms of accurate and easy definition bladder neck involvement and seminal vesicle invasion (Table **4.5**). In particular, when comparing the findings observed with the approach proposed here with those of the past when a more traditional approach was used, a 3 % increase of the microscopic involvement of the bladder neck and a 2 % increase in the microscopic involvement of the seminal vesicle have been seen [20].

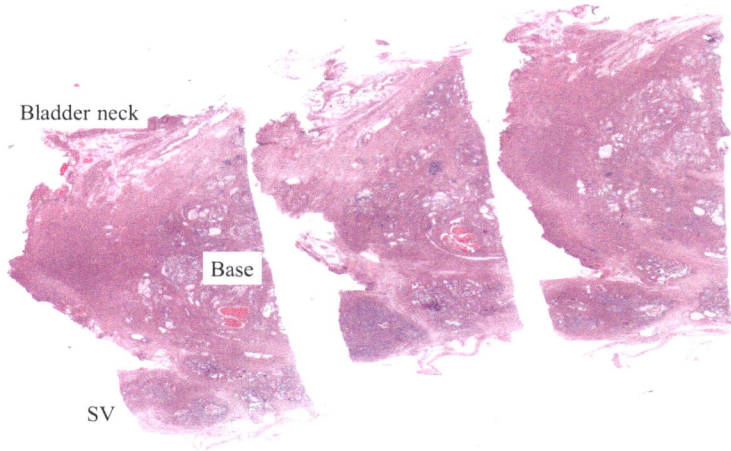

Fig. 4.5 Prostate base, including the bladder neck, and proximal part of the seminal vesicles examined with the whole mount technique

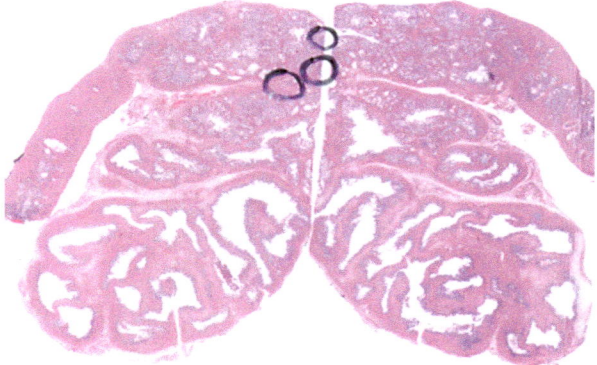

Fig. 4.6 The seminal vesicles examined with the whole mount technique. The *circle areas* represent small foci of cancer

Table 4.5 Advantages with the combined handling of prostate base/bladder neck and seminal vesicles in radical prostatectomy specimens

1. Microscopic involvement of the bladder neck, i.e. pT3a
2. Surgical margin status in the whole basal surface
3. Microscopic involvement of the seminal vesicle at the junction with the prostate
4. Types of cancer spread to the seminal vesicles and amount of cancer in the seminal vesicles
5. Minimal extraprostatic extension in the adipose tissue that surrounds the seminal vesicles and in the lateral pedicles

Conclusions

Handling of radical prostatectomy specimens is a challenging task for the pathologist. Prostate cancer is notoriously difficult to identify with the naked eye, the tumours are smaller but yet more multifocal than most other clinically diagnosed cancers and prostate cancer is very heterogeneous, both morphologically and genetically. Thus, these specimens need to be handled with great care and according to standardized protocols to enable accurate assessment of grade and stage.

References

1. Hall GS, Kramer CE, Epstein JI (1992) Evaluation of radical prostatectomy specimens. A comparative analysis of sampling methods. Am J Surg Pathol 16:315–324
2. Montironi R, Lopez Beltran A, Mazzucchelli R, Cheng L, Scarpelli M (2012) Handling of radical prostatectomy specimens: total embedding with large-format histology. Int J Breast Cancer 2012:6
3. Samaratunga H, Montironi R, True L, Epstein JI, Griffiths DF, Humphrey PA, van der Kwast T, Wheeler TM, Srigley JR, Delahunt B, Egevad L, ISUP Prostate Cancer Group (2011) International Society of Urological Pathology (ISUP) Consensus conference on handling and staging of radical prostatectomy specimens. Working group 1: specimen handling. Mod Pathol 24:6–15
4. Sehdev AE, Pan CC, Epstein JI (2001) Comparative analysis of sampling methods for grossing radical prostatectomy specimens for nonpalpable [stage T1c] prostatic adenocarcinoma. Hum Pathol 32:494–499
5. Montironi R, Lopez-Beltran A, Scarpelli M, Mazzucchelli R, Cheng L (2011) Handling of radical prostatectomy specimens: total embedding with whole mounts, with special reference to the Ancona experience. Histopathology 59:1006–1010
6. Berney D, Wheeler T, Grignon D et al (2011) International Society of Urological Pathology (ISUP) consensus conference on handling and staging of radical prostatectomy specimens: Working group 4: seminal vesicles and lymph nodes. Mod Pathol 24:39–47
7. Magi-Galluzzi C, Evans A, Delahunt B et al (2011) International Society of Urological Pathology (ISUP) consensus conference on handling and staging of radical prostatectomy specimens: Working group 3: extraprostatic extension, lymphovascular invasion and locally advanced disease. Mod Pathol 24:26–38
8. Tan PH, Cheng L, Srigley JR et al (2011) International Society of Urological Pathology (ISUP) consensus conference on handling and staging of radical prostatectomy specimens: Working group 5: surgical margins. Mod Pathol 24:48–57
9. van der Kwast T, Amin MB, Billis A et al (2011) International Society of Urological Pathology (ISUP) consensus conference on handling and staging of radical prostatectomy specimens: Working group 2: T2 sub-staging and prostate cancer volume. Mod Pathol 24:16–25
10. Kench JG, Clouston DR, Delprado W, Eade T, Ellis D, Horvath LG, Samaratunga H, Stahl J, Stapleton AM, Egevad L, Srigley JR, Delahunt B (2011) Prognostic factors in prostate cancer. Key elements in structured histopathology reporting of radical prostatectomy specimens. Pathology 43:410–419
11. Srigley JR, Humphrey PA, Amin MB, Chang SS, Egevad L, Epstein JI, Grignon DJ, McKiernan JM, Montironi R, Renshaw AA, Reuter VE, Wheeler TM, Members of the Cancer Committee, College of American Pathologists (2009) Protocol for the examination of specimens from patients with carcinoma of the prostate gland. Arch Pathol Lab Med 133:1568–1576

12. True LD (1994) Surgical pathology examination of the prostate gland. Practice survey by American Society of Clinical Pathologists. Am J Clin Pathol 102:572–579
13. Egevad L, Algaba F, Berney DM, Boccon-Gibod L, Griffiths DF, Lopez-Beltran A, Mikuz G, Varma M, Montironi R, European Network of Uropathology (2008) Handling and reporting of radical prostatectomy specimens in Europe: a web-based survey by the European Network of Uropathology (ENUP). Histopathology 53:333–339
14. Vainer B, Toft BG, Olsen KE, Jacobsen GK, Marcussen N (2011) Handling of radical prostatectomy specimens: total or partial embedding? Histopathology 58:211–216
15. Cohen MB, Soloway MS, Murphy WM (1994) Sampling of radical prostatectomy specimens. How much is adequate? Am J Clin Pathol 101:250–252
16. Mazzucchelli R, Barbisan F, Tagliabracci A, Lopez-Beltran A, Cheng L, Scarpelli M, Montironi R (2007) Search for residual prostate cancer on pT0 radical prostatectomy after positive biopsy. Virchows Arch 450:371–378
17. Montironi R, Cheng L, Lopez-Beltran A, Scarpelli M, Mazzucchelli R, Mikuz G, Kirkali Z, Montorsi F (2009) Stage pT0 in radical prostatectomy with no residual carcinoma and with a previous positive biopsy conveys a wrong message to clinicians and patients: why is cancer not present in the radical prostatectomy specimen? Eur Urol 56:272–274
18. Mazzucchelli R, Scarpelli M, Cheng L et al (2009) Pathology of prostate cancer and focal therapy ('male lumpectomy'). Anticancer Res 29:5155–5161
19. Montironi R, Cheng L, Lopez-Beltran A et al (2009) Joint appraisal of the radical prostatectomy specimen by the urologist and the uropathologist: together, we can do it better. Eur Urol 56:951–955
20. Montironi R, Cheng L, Lopez-Beltran A, Mazzucchelli R, Scarpelli M (2013) Combined handling of prostate base/bladder neck and seminal vesicles in radical prostatectomy specimens: our approach with the whole mount technique. Histopathology 63(3):431–435
21. Bostwick DG, Foster CS, Algaba F, Hutter RVP, Montironi R, Mostofi FK, Sakr W, Sesterhenn I (2000) Prostate tissue factors. In: Murphy G, Khoury S, Partin A, Denis L (eds) Prostate cancer. 2nd International consultation on prostate cancer. Plymbridge Distributors, Plymouth, UK, pp 162–201

The Dilemma of Early Diagnosis for a Clinically Relevant Prostate Cancer: The Role of Urologist

Susanna Cattarino and Mauro Ciccariello

5.1   Introduction

Cancer of the prostate (PCa) is now recognized as one of the most important medical problems facing the male population. Furthermore, PCa is currently the second most common cause of cancer death in men [1, 2]. Over the past decade, there has been a marked decline in PCa mortality corresponding to the introduction of Prostate-Specific Antigen (PSA) test as a screening tool (1986) [3]. PSA is a kallikrein-like serine protease produced almost exclusively by the epithelial cells of the prostate. The level of PSA as an independent variable is a better predictor of cancer than suspicious findings on digital rectal examination (DRE) or transrectal ultrasound (TRUS) [4]. Actually, there is no universally accepted cut-off for upper limit for PSA level. The level of *PSA* is a continuous parameter: the higher the value, the more likely is the existence of PCa. The findings that many men may harbour PCa despite low levels of serum PSA have been underscored by results from US Prevention study [5]. Despite it is well recognized as a good marker for PCa risk by the medical community, it is still considered an "imperfect" marker for the following reasons:

- It is organ specific but not cancer specific.
- PSA has a limited specificity and sensitivity in determining the presence of PCa, especially in the total PSA range between 2 and 10 ng/ml ("The grey zone") [6].
- It cannot well distinguish indolent and lethal cancers; some men have an aggressive form of PCa for which screening might be helpful, but many have a low-grade cancer that would never progress to cause serious illness during a man's lifetime and their detection could bring an overtreatment.

There is still no absolute proof that PSA screening reduces mortality due to PCa [7]. Two large, prospective, randomized trials on PCa *screening*, conducted in 2009, published conflicting results. The Prostate, Lung, Colorectal and Ovarian

S. Cattarino (✉) • M. Ciccariello
Department of Urology, University Sapienza Rome, Viale del Policninico 155, Rome 00161, Italy
e-mail: Susanna.cattarino@uniroma1.it; Mauro.ciccariello@uniroma1.it

V. Gentile et al. (eds.), *Multidisciplinary Management of Prostate Cancer*,
DOI 10.1007/978-3-319-04385-2_5, © Springer International Publishing Switzerland 2014

(PLCO) Cancer Screening trial [8] concluded that PCa-related mortality was very low and not significantly different between the group that received annual screening with PSA and the control group. The incidence of death per 10,000 person-year was 2.0 (50 deaths) in the screened group and 1.7 (44 deaths) in the control group (RR: 1.13). The European Randomized Study of Screening for Prostate Cancer (ERSPC) [9] investigators concluded that PSA-based screening reduced the rate of deaths from PCa by 20 % but was associated with a high risk of overdiagnosis. Based on these results, the major urological societies conclude that, at present, widespread mass screening for PCa is not appropriate.

The aim of this section is to summarize the new biomarkers and modern clinical approaches based on international published data that can improve PSA specificity and help the dilemma of the urologist for an early diagnosis of PCa.

5.2   PSA Free

The measurement of PSA suffers from a lack of specificity because various benign prostatic conditions can also lead to increased serum PSA. The immunologically measurable PSA in serum is present in the non-complexed 33-kDa form, called free PSA "fPSA" and in a complex one, called "cPSA", primarily with the serum protease inhibitor alpha1antichymotrypsin (ACT). Total PSA "tPSA" is equal to *fPSA + cPSA*. The proportion or ratio of fPSA to tPSA in serum (%fPSA) has been demonstrated to significantly improve the discrimination of PCa from benign conditions, particularly in patients with tPSA concentrations in 2–10 ng/ml. A meta-analysis containing 41 studies [10] reveals an area under the curve (AUC) for %fPSA of 0.70 for all PSA levels, decreasing to 0.68 in the "grey zone". A test cut-off of 20 % would lead to 92 % sensitivity and 23 % specificity. Positive likelihood ratios range from 1.0 to 4.0 at %fPSA of 15 % or less. Roddam et al. [11] demonstrated a sensitivity of 95 % and a specificity of 18 % of %fPSA in 4–10 ng/ml tPSA range and an AUC of 66.7 % for detecting PCa in men with tPSA <4 ng/ml.

5.3   PSA Kinetics

PSA kinetics, in the form of *PSA velocity*, defined as an absolute annual increase in serum PSA and *PSA doubling time*, which measures the exponent increase of serum PSA overtime may have a prognostic role in patients curatively treated with surgery or radiation therapy [12], but they have limited use in the diagnosis of PCa. Optimal time intervals for calculation and optimal thresholds are still to be determined.

5.4   proPSA and Derivatives

In the tPSA range between 2 and 10 ng/ml, no single biomarker can accurately predict the result of an initial biopsy. Pro or precursor forms of PSA have emerged as potentially important diagnostic serum markers for PCa detection. *proPSA* is the precursor form of PSA and contains a 7 amino acid pro leader peptide. Additional truncated forms of proPSA exist in serum, primarily those with leader sequences of 5, 4 and 2 amino acids. Cleavage of the leader sequences by human kallikrein 2 (hkr) and trypsin to activate PSA decreases with decreasing size of the propeptide leader sequence with [−2] proPSA resistant to activation. [−2] proPSA is the most relevant form in tumour extracts and immunohistochemically stains cancer cells more strongly than benign cells [13]. The [−2] proPSA form and the other proPSA forms have been studied individually and in combination and suggest a role for these molecular forms of PSA in the early detection of PCa [14] as well as in discriminating between indolent and lethal cancers [15, 16]. In a retrospective study of Sokoll et al. [17] PSA, %fPSA, [−2]proPSA %[−2]proPSA were calculated in 89 men selected for prostate biopsy in the tPSA range between 2 and 10 ng/ml. Of the PSA derivatives, *%[−2]proPSA* had the greatest AUC of 0.73 followed by [−2] proPSA with an AUC of 0.65 while the AUC for %fPSA was 0.53. At a sensitivity of 90 % corresponding specificity was 18 % for %fPSA and 41 % for %[−2] proPSA, respectively. In an observational prospective study, Guazzoni et al. [16] investigated the accuracy of [−2]proPSA, %[−2] proPSA and the *Prostate Health Index* $\left(\text{p2PSA/fPSA} \times \sqrt{\text{TPSA}}\right)$ (phi) between patients with or without PCa in the tPSA range between 2.0 and 10 ng/ml. In an univariate accuracy analysis, %[−2] proPSA (AUC: 75.7 %) and phi (AUC: 75.6 %) were the most accurate predictors and significantly outperformed %fPSA (AUC: 57.9 %) and PSA density (AUC: 60.8 %) in the prediction of PCa at biopsy. Specifically, %[−2]proPSA and phi were 23 % more accurate than tPSA in detecting patients with PCa. Similarly, at 90 % specificity, the sensitivity of phi (42 %) and of %[−2]proPSA (38 %) were significantly higher than those of tPSA (51 %), %fPSA (20.0 %) and PSA density (26.5 %). The inclusion of %[−2]proPSA or phi in a multivariate logistic regression model resulted in a 10 % and 11 % increase of its predictive accuracy, respectively. They demonstrated that the implementation of %[−2]proPSA and phi in clinical practice may significantly increase our ability to detect PCa, lowering the number of unnecessary biopsy. Data from the two studies [16, 17] are summarized in Table 5.1. It also defined to date, established clinical parameters used in PCa setting, such as PSA, DRE and Gleason score at biopsy often fail to accurately predict PCa aggressiveness. Consequently, PSA isoforms and its derivatives have been proposed to help the physicians in recognizing indolent and lethal cancers optimizing the decision-making process. Sokoll et al. [18] observed a direct relationship between [−2]pPSA and %[−2]proPSA and Gleason score in men with tPSA levels between 2 and 10 ng/ml. In fact, [−2]proPSA and %[−2]proPSA were significantly higher ([−2]proPSA: 12.0 VS. 8 pg/ml, $p < 0.001$; %[−2]pPSA: 1.66 % VS. 1.40 %, $p = 0.03$) in men with significant disease compared with men

Table 5.1 Comparison of outcomes from the Sokoll (2008) and Guazzoni (2011) studies

Studies	PSA and PSA derivatives studied	Study population	Number of patients	AUC	Sensitivity at 90 % specificity, %
Sokoll et al. J Urol (2008)	tPSA %fPSA [−2]proPSA %[−2]proPSA	No prior biopsy 2–10 ng/ml PSA range	89 men	0.52 0.53 0.65 0.73	18 41
Guazzoni et al. Eur Urol (2011)	tPSA %fPSA [−2]proPSA %[−2]proPSA phi index	Negative DRE 2–10 ng/ml PSA range	268 men	0.53 0.58 0.59 0.76 0.76	5.1 20.0 38.8 42.9

with insignificant disease, according to Epstein Criteria [19]. Similarly, results were shown by Guazzoni et al. [16] who confirmed a direct relationship between [−2] proPSA derivatives and PCa aggressiveness. %[−2]proPSA and phi represented the most accurate predictors of PCa with a *Gleason score* >7, outperforming patient age and %fPSA. Moreover, the same authors [20] found that [−2]proPSA and its derivatives are predictors of PCa characteristics at final pathology after radical prostatectomy (RP). On univariate analyses, %[−2]proPSA and phi emerged as the most accurate predictors of pT3 disease and pathologic Gleason sum ≥7. On multivariate analysis, the inclusion of %[−2]proPSA or phi increased their accuracy in predicting the pathological outcomes from 2.4 % to 6 %. The PRO-PSA Multicentric European Study, the Prometheus project resumed all this data [21]:

• [−2]proPSA (AUC: 0.733) and phi (AUC: 0.733) are more accurate than tPSA, fPSA and %fPSA in predicting PCa.
• Consideration of %[−2]proPSA and phi results in the avoidance of several unnecessary biopsies.
• [−2]proPSA and derivatives correlate with cancer aggressiveness.

They finally suggest to adopt these biomarkers in *preoperative counselling* for patients with clinically localized PCa in order to offer the best primary treatment, including active surveillance, RP, radiotherapy and focal therapy. Limits of these PSA derivatives might be summarized:

• Lack of standardization.
• The need to use them in association with PSA in a specific range (2–10 ng/ml).
• A total PSA might be influenced by benign conditions or medical treatment.
• No definition of an ideal cut-off.

Further studies in the form of large multicentre, prospective trials are required to evaluate the true clinical applicability.

Table 5.2 PCA3 characteristics

Setting	Outcomes of PCA3
Detection of PCa	Van Gils et al.: Sensitivity: 61 %, Specificity: 80 %, AUC: 0.70
Patients with prior negative biopsy	Diagnostic accuracy > %fPSA and not depend on the number of previous biopsies
PCa characterization	PCA3 > in GS > 7 PCA3 < in tumour volume <0.5 and insignificant tumour
Selection of patients for active survival	PCA3 good predictor in selection of patient with tumour volume < 0.5 and insignificant tumour
PCa calculator risk	PCA3 + PSA + DRE + age + race + prior biopsy + prostate biopsy: PCa RISK

5.5 PCA3

It has been shown that PSA performance in detecting PCa can be improved by the use of a new biomarker *PCA3*. Firstly described by Bussemakers et al. [22] PCA3 is a prostate-specific non-coding RNA which is highly over-expressed in more than 95 % of primary prostate tumours, with a median 66-fold up-regulation compared with adjacent non-cancer prostate tissue [22, 23]. The specificity of this marker for PCa has been confirmed by its lack of expression in other types of human tumours [23]. PCA3 has been demonstrated that might be helpful in different *setting* of patients: first diagnosis, prior negative biopsy, characterization of tumour, selection of patients for active surveillance and to calculate the risk of PCa (Table 5.2). Data from recent studies showed that PCA3 sensitivity ranges from 47 % to 69 %, specificity ranges from 66 % to 83 %, PPV ranges from 59 % to 97.4 %, NPV ranges from 87.7% to 98 % and AUC ranges from 0.65 to 0.74 [24]. European and American repeat biopsy studies have provided evidence that PCA3 values can add specificity to a diagnostic algorithm for PCa in men with previous negative biopsy. Haese et al. [25] showed that the PCA3 score had a greater diagnostic accuracy with a cut-off of 35 than %fPSA with a cut-off of 25 % and the diagnostic accuracy of the PCA3 assay is independent of the number of previous negative biopsies and of serum total PSA level. Emerging data are now available on the relationship between PCA3 and PCa features. In the study of Auprich et al. [26], PCA3 score was correlated with five distinct pathologic end points: low volume disease (<0.5 ml), insignificant PCa, extracapsular invasion (ECE), seminal vesicle invasion (SVI) and aggressive disease defined as Gleason sum >7. PCA3 scores were significantly lower in low-volume disease and insignificant PCa ($p \leq 0.001$) but not significantly elevated in pathologically confirmed ECE ($p = 0.4$) or SVI ($p = 0.5$). Higher PCA3 scores were associated with aggressive disease ($p < 0.001$). PCA3 score may be useful also to improve the selection of patients for active surveillance (AS) in addition to the current criteria. Ploussard et al. [27] revealed that PCA3 is independently associated with small volume disease (<0.5 ml) ($p < 0.001$) and pathologically confirmed insignificant PCa. The risk of having cancer ≥ 0.5 ml and a significant PCa was increased threefold in men with a PCA3 score ≥ 25 compared with men with a PCA3 score <25. In a multivariate analysis, taking into account other AS criteria (biopsy criteria, PSA density and Magnetic Resonance Imaging findings), a high PCA3 score (≥ 25) was an important predictive factor for tumour volume >0.5 (OR: 5.4, $p = 0.010$) and a significant PCa (OR: 12.7, $p = 0.003$). Recent data [28] suggest that the new biomarker PCA3 can be successfully incorporated into clinical tools for risk assessment, like Prostate Cancer Prevention Trial risk calculator (PCPT). Since its publication in 2006, the PCPT calculator combined six risk factors (PSA, DRE, age, race, history of biopsy and prostate biopsy) for PCa. Ankerst et al. [28] demonstrated that when PCA3 is incorporated into the PCPT risk calculator, the diagnostic accuracy significantly improved. On the basis of these summarized results, European guidelines recommend to use the PCA3 score together with PSA and other clinical risk factors in a nomogram or other risk stratification tools to make a decision with regard to first or repeat biopsy.

5.6   PSA and 5α Reductase Inhibitors

At this point of the discussion, readers should clearly understand how much it is important for a marker to be chosen by the urologist to discriminate the indolent from the aggressive PCa in order to choose which to treat and avoid overdiagnosis and overtreatment. The major helping came from the use of *5α reductase inhibitors* (5ARI) in patients at risk of PCa. The 5ARI, widely utilized for the treatment of BPH, block the conversion of testosterone to dihydrotestosterone inhibiting the enzyme 5α reductase. Finasteride inhibits selectively the type 2 isoform of 5α reductase; dutasteride is a dual inhibitor of the type 1 and 2 isoforms of the enzyme. The rationale for the use of 5ARI in the detection of PCa is based on the fact that they suppress PSA production related to benign prostatic hyperplasia (BPH) progression, so, consequently, they significantly impact the validity of PSA as a marker for PCa. Two recent and large clinical trials demonstrated that the use of 5α reductase inhibitors can prevent PCa: The Reduction by Dutasteride of Prostate Cancer Events (*REDUCE*) [29] and the Prostate Cancer Prevention Trial (*PCPT*) [30]. The REDUCE study [29] compared dutasteride, at dose of 0.5 mg daily, with placebo in men with PSA level of 2.5 to 10 ng/ml and a prior negative prostate biopsy. The end points were PCa detection on biopsy after 2 and 4 years of treatment and Gleason score at biopsy, the presence of pre-neoplastic lesions and other end points related to BPH. Andriole et al. concluded that dutasteride reduced the risk of incident PCa detected on biopsy: 659/3,305 (19.9 %) in the treated group and 858/3,424 (25 %) in the placebo group had PCa. *Dutasteride* was associated with a relative risk reduction of 22.8 % (95 % CI, 15.2–29.8, $p < 0.001$). They observed a significant difference between the two groups according to Gleason score at biopsy: 437 tumours in the treated group and 617 in control group were Gleason score of 5 to 6. Other results were: a reduction of the number of cases of pre-neoplastic lesions in the dutasteride group and an improvement of many outcomes related to BPH. The PCPT [30] was designed to reduce the prevalence

Table 5.3 Comparison of results from the REDUCE and PCPT studies

Outcome Dutasteride or Finasteride arm versus Placebo arm P value	REDUCE	PCPT
Number of patients	3,305 3,424	4,579 5,112
PCa	659/3,305 (19 %) 858/3,424 (25 %) $p < 0.001$	695/4,579 (15.2 %) 1,111/5,112 (21.7 %) $p < 0.001$
Gleason score GS (5 or 6)/GS ≥ 7	437/3,299 (13.2 %) 617/3,407 (18.1 %) $p < 0001$	264/686 (38.5 %) 240/1,100 (21.8 %) $p = 0.03$
Gleason score GS (7–10)/GS ≥ 8	220/3,299 (6.7 %) 233/3,407 (6.8 %) $p = 0.81$	81/686 (11.8 %) 55/1,100 (5 %) $p = 0.71$

of PCa after 7 years of treatment. They concluded that the prevalence of PCa was reduced by 24.8 % in the finasteride group compared with the placebo group and that the absolute numbers of high-grade tumours (GS ≥ 7) were higher in the treated group (280/757, 37 %) than in placebo group (237/1,068, 22.2 %). Later, they also examined the impact of finasteride on the sensitivity and AUC of PSA for detecting PCa, in particular high-grade PCa (GS ≥ 7). The sensitivities of PSA were uniformly greater in the *finasteride* group than in the placebo group: 37.8 % (95 % CI = 34.2–41.4), 53.0 % (95 % CI = 47.0–59.0) and 64.2 % (95 % CI = 53.8–74.6) for PCa, Gleason grade 7 or higher and Gleason grade 8 or higher disease, respectively in the finasteride arm compared with 24.0 % (95 % CI = 21.5–26.5), 39.2 % (95 % CI = 33.0–45.4) and 49.1 % (95 % CI = 35.9–62.3), respectively, in the placebo arm. Compared data of these two trials are summarized in Table 5.3.

Indeed, this effect of finasteride on the sensitivity of PSA may have been at least in part responsible for the increased detection of high-grade disease. Consequently, the phenomenon (higher sensitivity for cancer detection and higher risk of high-grade disease with higher PSA in finasteride treatment) would be expected to artificially increase high-grade cancer detection in men treated with finasteride with the risk of limiting the potential public health benefit of the drug [31]. The explanation is that if finasteride treatment would cause a greatest fall in PSA levels in men with BPH, the men with persistently higher PSA levels in treated group would therefore be more likely to have cancer. Moreover, higher PSA levels are also more likely to reflect the presence of high-grade cancer. For this reason, it is very important to clarify the adjustments that should be made regarding PSA levels to ensure that 5ARI therapy is applied and the usefulness of PSA as a PCa marker is maintained.

Andriole et al. [32] in their study wanted to assess whether *dutasteride* enhances the usefulness of PSA for the diagnosis of clinically significant PCa based on data from the REDUCE trial. They observed that final PSA before biopsy and the change from month 6 to final PSA performed better for the diagnosis of Gleason score 7–10 tumours in men who received dutasteride VS. placebo. Increases in PSA were associated with higher likelihood of biopsy detectable, Gleason score 7–10 and clinically significant tumours. Finally, they also observed that percentage decreases in PSA from baseline to month 6 in the dutasteride group did not predict PCa overall or the likelihood of PC. Also, the results of Marberger et al. [33] based on the REDUCE data supported the idea that PSA kinetics accurately reflect the biology of PCa in men receiving dutasteride. By suppressing PSA from benign prostatic tissue and *indolent cancers*, subsequent rises in PSA levels after nadir may reflect growth that is not controlled by dutasteride. This may suggest that in men taking dutasteride, even high-grade cancers without a rising PSA are behaving indolently. A small rise that does not progress over time might not be meaningful and one needs to approach a single nadir value with the same approach as a single rise from a supposed *nadir*. Very small (0.1–0.2 ng/ml) rises in PSA may be particularly difficult to interpret. Thus, some studies [34] have some recommendation for the choice of PSA rise for making biopsy in men receiving treatment. The original observation that finasteride decreased serum PSA by approximately 50 % within 6 months lead to the recommendation that the *doubled PSA* should be used for the clinical decision in men receiving 5ARI therapy [35]. Marks et al. [34] proposed that a PSA increase from nadir of 0.3 ng/ml or greater in treated patients could represent a better alternative to the doubling rule for monitoring PSA in treated patients. They demonstrated that an increase in PSA of 0.3 ng/ml from nadir as a trigger for *biopsy* maintains 71 % of sensitivity for PCa in men receiving dutasteride with 60 % of specificity which is similar to the specificity of a 4.0 ng/ml PSA cut-off with placebo.

Based on data from these two trials we can resume that:

- The extent of the PSA level decrease in the first 6 months does not predict the diagnosis of PCa.
- Patients receiving dutasteride/finasteride should have a new PSA baseline established after 6 months of treatment.
- Any confirmed increase from lowest PSA level in dutasteride/finasteride treatment may signal the presence of PCa, particularly *high grade*.
- The treatment with dutasteride/finasteride does not interfere with the use of PSA as a tool to assist the diagnosis of PCa.
- For men who are concerned about PCa (familial disease, abnormal PSA, increased PSA velocity/doubling time), it may be appropriate to discuss chemoprevention with finasteride/dutasteride.
- It is important to highlight both the benefits and potential side effects associated with long-term treatment with finasteride/dutasteride.

Freedland in his editorial [36] answers to some conflicting questions and tries to assist the clinicians in everyday practice in three different situations: men on 5ARI treatment with a consistently rising PSA are recommended to repeat a biopsy; men on 5ARI treatment with a stable or declining PSA are not recommended to repeat biopsy and men on 5ARI treatment with a prior negative biopsy at very low-risk PSA (<0.5 ml) are not recommended to repeat biopsy because it will be missed some high-grade cancer although 99 % of these men will not have high-grade cancers. It can be affirmed that 5ARI therapy can reduce the number of men undergoing *"unnecessary biopsy"*.

5.7 Indication for Prostate Biopsy and Limits of Prostate Biopsy

After a correct use of biomarkers in the detection of PCa, the second step in the early diagnosis of PCa is its histological confirmation at prostate biopsy (PBx). Although the random TRUS-guided biopsy remains the gold standard for PCa detection, it has been reported to miss up to 30 % of cancers. Over the last few years, more efficient biopsy schemes for detecting PCa have been proposed. After the initial introduction of the *sextant PBx* technique proposed by Hodge [37] that represented the standard method for many years, more extended PBx schemes resulted in higher cancer detection rate. As defined by the National Comprehensive Cancer Network, an extended prostate biopsy (EPBx) is essentially a sextant template with at least four additional cores from the lateral peripheral zone, that are the sites at which PCa is most likely to be located. It has been reported that laterally directed biopsies, yield about a 25 % increase in the ability to detect PCa [38–40] without significant morbidity. However, it still remains controversial defining the optimal number of cores and actual limits of PBx can be clearly summarized. Biopsy strategies with an increased number of cores (*"saturation biopsy"*, ≥24) have been suggested to reduce false-negative rate, but the incidence of PCa detected with this technique is between 30 % and 43 % and depends on the number of cores sampled. Men with persistently elevated serum PSA levels after a negative first random PBx could represent the main target of saturation biopsy. Simply repeated random biopsies in patients with persistently increasing serum PSA show gradually decreasing results as the number of *re-biopsy* rounds increases, evolving from a 23 % cancer detection rate at the first round to a 17.6 %, 11.7 %, 8.7 % and 0 % at the 2nd, 3rd, 4th and 5th round, respectively [41]. At the moment, no clear criteria indicate when to perform a re-biopsy in patients with persistently elevated levels of PSA with prior negative PBx. Today, a PBx is not only a method to diagnose PCa, but it correlated with other parameters including tumour volume and Gleason score, that may have an impact on clinical decision-making. It is well known that prostate volume is one of the factors that may influence the prediction of cancer at first biopsy and that a significant inverse relationship exists between the cancer detection rate and prostate volume [42]. Recently, it was shown that 14-core biopsies are superior to 8-core biopsies for patients with *prostate volume* of 30–40 cc. A core number > 14 may be needed to detect cancer for prostate volumes >40 cc [43]. It is very important to obtain a diagnosis as close as possible to the real pathological characteristics of prostate tumour in order to plan the optimal therapeutic strategy, even more important for those patients candidates for radiotherapy, in which the only data come from PBx. Different studies have demonstrated that the ability of EPBx to predict the final Gleason score is higher [44] than the ability of standard sextant biopsy (28–48 %) [44, 45]. Different authors [46, 47] have

Table 5.4 PSA performance for a cut-off of 2.5 ng/ml for early diagnosis of PC in the REDUCE and PCPT studies

	REDUCE		PCPT	
PSA	Dutasteride group	Placebo group	Finasteride group	Placebo group
Sensitivity	0.805	0.996	0.138	0.428
Specificity	0.434	0.044	0.981	0.800
PPV	0.092	0.071		
NPV	0.969	0.993		

demonstrated that, with more cores, the risk of significant *"upgrading"* at final pathology after RP decreases because of higher sampling density and more accurate pathologic biopsy evaluation. A possible explanation of this phenomenon of upgrading is believed to be attributed to a greater difficulty in correctly determining the Gleason PBx in high volume gland, maintaining a sextant scheme. We can find a significant confirmation in the results of the PCPT [30] where the high number of high-grade tumours observed at biopsy in the finasteride arm compared with placebo would be due to artefacts secondary to changes in prostate volume and not to an inductive effect of finasteride on the development of high-grade tumours. The reduction of prostate volume in the active treatment arm would allow a better definition of the biopsy Gleason thereby significantly reducing the phenomenon of "upgrading". Predictive *nomograms* [48] have been developed as prognostic models capable of predicting the probability of significant upgrading. Nowadays, PBx represents the diagnostic method to monitoring patients selected for active surveillance; also for this reason, predictive nomograms have been necessary as prognostic models capable of defining the morphologic characterisation of PCa (Table 5.4).

Conclusions

In conclusions, we can affirm that the urological community has to work hard to find a "better" marker or medical approach that can help the clinicians in the early diagnosis of PCa and that can finally discriminate the tumour that will or will not affect a man during his natural lifetime. Moreover, we need for a more sensitive and accurate imaging modality to direct biopsy and to detect early PCa.

References

1. Boyle P, Ferlay J (2005) Cancer incidence and mortality in Europe 2004. Ann Oncol 16 (3):481–488
2. Jemal A, Siegel R, Ward E et al (2008) Cancer statistics, 2008. CA Cancer J Clin 58(2):71–96
3. Collin SM, Martin RM, Metcalfe C et al (2008) Prostate-cancer mortality in the USA and UK in 1975–2004: an ecological study. Lancet Oncol 9(5):445–452
4. Catalona WJ, Richie JP, Ahmann FR et al (1994) Comparison of digital rectal examination and serum prostate specific antigen in the early detection of prostate cancer: results of a multicenter clinical trial of 6,630 men. J Urol 151(5):1283–1290

5. Thompson IM, Pauler DK, Goodman PJ et al (2004) Prevalence of prostate cancer among men with a prostate-specific antigen level < or =4.0 ng per milliliter. N Engl J Med 350(22):2239–2246
6. Schroder FH, Roobol MJ (2009) Defining the optimal prostate-specific antigen threshold for the diagnosis of prostate cancer. Curr Opin Urol 19:227–231
7. Ilic D, O'Connor D, Green S et al (2007) Screening for prostate cancer: a Cochrane systematic review. Cancer Causes Control 18(3):279–285
8. Andriole GL, Crawford ED, Grubb RL et al (2009) Mortality results from a randomized prostate-cancer screening trial. N Engl J Med 360:1310–1319
9. Schröder FH, Hugosson J, Roobol MJ et al (2009) Screening and prostate-cancer mortality in a randomized European study. N Engl J Med 360:1320–1328
10. Lee R, Localio AR, Armstrong K, Free PSA Study Group et al (2006) A meta-analysis of the performance characteristics of the free prostate-specific antigen test. Urology 67(4):762–768
11. Roddam AW, Duffy MJ, Hamdy FC et al (2005) Use of prostate-specific antigen (PSA) isoforms for the detection of prostate cancer in men with a PSA level of 2–10 ng/ml: systematic review and meta-analysis. Eur Urol 48:386–399
12. Maffezzini M, Bossi A, Collette L (2007) Implications of prostate-specific antigen doubling time as indicator of failure after surgery or radiation therapy for prostate cancer. Eur Urol 51 (3):605–613, Discussion 613
13. Chan TY, Mikolajczyk SD, Lecksell K et al (2003) Immunohistochemical staining of prostate cancer with monoclonal antibodies to the precursor of prostate-specific antigen. Urology 62 (1):177–181
14. Mikolajczyk SD, Catalona WJ, Evans CL et al (2004) Proenzyme forms of prostate-specific antigen in serum improve the detection of prostate cancer. Clin Chem 50:1017
15. Catalona WJ, Bartsch G, Rittenhouse HG et al (2004) Serum proprostate specific antigen preferentially detects aggressive prostate cancers in men with 2 to 4 ng/ml prostate specific antigen. J Urol 171:2239
16. Guazzoni G, Nava L, Lazzeri M et al (2011) Prostate-specific antigen (PSA) isoform p2PSA significantly improves the prediction of prostate cancer at initial extended prostate biopsies in patients with total PSA between 2.0 and 10 ng/ml: results of a prospective study in a clinical setting. Eur Urol 60(2):214–222
17. Sokoll LJ, Wang Y, Feng Z et al (2008) [-2]proenzyme prostate specific antigen for prostate cancer detection: a national cancer institute early detection research network validation study. J Urol 180(2):539–543
18. Sokoll LJ, Sanda MG, Feng Z et al (2010) A prospective, multicenter, national cancer institute early detection research network study of [-2]proPSA: improving prostate cancer detection and correlating with cancer aggressiveness. Cancer Epidemiol Biomarkers Prev 19:1193–1200
19. Epstein J, Walsh P, Carmichael M et al (1994) Pathologic and clinical findings to predict tumor extent of nonpalpable (stage T1c) prostate cancer. JAMA 27:368–374
20. Guazzoni G, Lazzeri M, Nava L et al (2012) Preoperative prostate-specific antigen isoform p2PSA and its derivatives, %p2PSA and prostate health index, predict pathologic outcomes in patients undergoing radical prostatectomy for prostate cancer. Eur Urol 61(3):455–466
21. Lazzeri M, Haese A, Abrate A et al (2013) Clinical performance of serum prostate-specific antigen isoform [-2]proPSA (p2PSA) and its derivatives, %p2PSA and the prostate health index (PHI), in men with a family history of prostate cancer: results from a multicentre European study, the PROMEtheuS project. BJU Int 112(3):313–321
22. de Kok JB, Verhaegh GW, Roelofs RW et al (2002) DD3(PCA3), a very sensitive and specific marker to detect prostate tumors. Cancer Res 62:2695–2698
23. Hessels D, Klein Gunnewiek JM, van Oort I et al (2003) DD3(PCA3)-based molecular urine analysis for the diagnosis of prostate cancer. Eur Urol 44:8–15
24. Roobol MJ, Schröder FH, van Leeuwen P et al (2010) Performance of the prostate cancer antigen 3 (PCA3) gene and prostate-specific antigen in prescreened men: exploring the value of PCA3 for a first-line diagnostic test. Eur Urol 58(4):475–481

25. Haese A, de la Taille A, van Poppel H et al (2008) Clinical utility of the PCA3 urine assay in European men scheduled for repeat biopsy. Eur Urol 54(5):1081–1088
26. Auprich M, Chun FK, Ward JF et al (2011) Critical assessment of preoperative urinary prostate cancer antigen 3 on the accuracy of prostate cancer staging. Eur Urol 59(1):96–105
27. Ploussard G, Durand X, Xylinas E et al (2011) Prostate cancer antigen 3 score accurately predicts tumour volume and might help in selecting prostate cancer patients for active surveillance. Eur Urol 59(3):422–429
28. Ankerst DP, Groskopf J, Day JR et al (2008) Predicting prostate cancer risk through incorporation of prostate cancer gene 3. J Urol 180:1303–1308
29. Andriole GL, Bostwick DG, Brawley OW et al (2010) Effect of dutasteride on the risk of prostate cancer. N Engl J Med 362(13):1192–1202
30. Thompson IM, Goodman PJ, Tangen CM et al (2003) The influence of finasteride on the development of prostate cancer. N Engl J Med 349:215–224
31. Thompson IM, Chi C, Ankerst DP et al (2006) Effect of finasteride on the sensitivity of PSA for detecting prostate cancer. J Natl Cancer Inst 98(16):1128–33
32. Andriole GL, Bostwick D, Brawley OW et al (2011) The effect of dutasteride on the usefulness of prostate specific antigen for the diagnosis of high grade and clinically relevant prostate cancer in men with a previous negative biopsy: results from the REDUCE study. J Urol 185 (1):126–131
33. Marberger M, Freedland SJ, Andriole GL et al (2012) Usefulness of prostate-specific antigen (PSA) rise as a marker of prostate cancer in men treated with dutasteride: lessons from the REDUCE study. BJU Int 109(8):1162–1169
34. Marks LS, Andriole GL, Fitzpatrick JM et al (2006) The interpretation of serum prostate specific antigen in men receiving 5alpha-reductase inhibitors: a review and clinical recommendations. J Urol 176(3):868–874
35. Gormley GJ, Stoner E, Bruskewitz RC et al (1992) The effect of finasteride in men with benign prostatic hyperplasia. The Finasteride Study Group. N Engl J Med 327:1185–1191
36. Freedland SJ, Andriole GL (2011) Making an imperfect marker better. Eur Urol 59(2):194–196
37. Hodge KK, McNeal JE, Terris MK et al (1989) Random systematic versus directed ultrasound guided transrectal core biopsies of the prostate. J Urol 142(1):71–74
38. Meng MV, Franks JH, Presti JC Jr et al (2003) The utility of apical anterior horn biopsies in prostate cancer detection. Urol Oncol 21:361–365
39. De la Taille A, Antiphon P, Salomon L et al (2003) Prospective evaluation of a 21-sample needle biopsy procedure designed to improve the prostate cancer detection rate. Urology 61:1181–1186
40. Eskew LA, Bare RL, McCullough DL (1997) Systematic 5 region prostate biopsy is superior to sextant method for diagnosing carcinoma of the prostate. J Urol 157:199–202
41. Zackrisson B, Aus G, Bergdahl S et al (2004) The risk of findings focal cancer (less than 3 mm) remains high on re-biopsy of patients with persistently increased prostate specific antigen but the clinical significance is questionable. J Urol 171:1500–1503
42. Djavan B (2006) Prostate biopsies and Vienna nomograms. Eur Urol Suppl 5:500–510
43. Inahara M, Suzuki H, Kojima S et al (2006) Improved prostate cancer detection using systematic 14-core biopsy for large prostate glands with normal digital rectal examination findings. Urology 68:815–819
44. San Francisco IF, DeWolf WC, Rosen S, Upton M, Olumi AF (2003) Extended prostate needle biopsy improves concordance of Gleason grading between prostate needle biopsy and radical prostatectomy. J Urol 169:136–140
45. King CR, McNeal JE, Gill H et al (2004) Extended prostate biopsy scheme improves reliability of Gleason grading: implications for radiotherapy patients. Int J Radiat Oncol Biol Phys 59:386–391
46. King CR, Patel DA, Terris MK (2005) Prostate biopsy volume indices do not predict for significant Gleason upgrading. Am J Clin Oncol 28:125–129

47. Freedland SJ, Kane CJ, Amling CL, SEARCH Database Study Group et al (2007) Upgrading and downgrading of prostate needle biopsy specimens: risk factors and clinical implications. Urology 69:495–499
48. Chun FK, Briganti A, Shariat SF et al (2006) Significant upgrading affects a third of men diagnosed with prostate cancer: predictive nomogram and internal validation. BJU Int 98:329–334

Modern Imaging in the Initial Diagnosis: The Role of the Radiologist in an MDT

Flavio Barchetti, Valerio Forte, Maria Giulia Bernieri, and Valeria Panebianco

6.1 Introduction

Despite recent advances in prostate cancer (PC) detection and treatment, PC continues to be one of the leading causes of cancer-related mortality in men. Thus, accurate diagnosis and appropriate treatment are crucial. The detection of PC is traditionally based on digital rectal examination (DRE), clinical stage and the measurement of serum prostate-specific antigen (PSA), followed by transrectal ultrasound (TRUS)-guided biopsies. However, PSA has a poor specificity and low predictive value, and therefore, many biopsies may be tumour negative. Moreover, with the current biopsy scheme, only a small portion of the prostate gland is sampled, with the risk of missing a significant lesion. Random TRUS-guided biopsy misses about 30 % of cancerous lesions, 23 % of which are high risk of PC [1]. Nowadays, there is a real need for clinicians to base therapeutic decisions not only on PSA serum level, DRE and TRUS-biopsy results, but also on imaging findings. In recent years, various imaging modalities have been developed to improve diagnosis, staging and localisation of early-stage PC. Conventional TRUS is mainly used to guide prostate biopsy. Contrast-enhanced US (CEUS) is based on the assumption that PC tissue is hypervascularised and might be better identified after intravenous injection of a microbubble contrast agent. Real-time elastography (RTE) seems to have higher sensitivity (Se), specificity (Spe) and positive predictive value (PPV) than conventional TRUS. However, the method still awaits prospective validation.

F. Barchetti • V. Forte • M.G. Bernieri
Department of Radiological Sciences, Oncology and Pathology, University of Rome, Viale Del Policlinico 155, Rome 00161, Italy, Lazio
e-mail: flavio.barchetti@live.it

V. Panebianco (✉)
Department of Radiological Sciences, Oncology & Pathology, Sapienza University, Policlinico Umberto I, Viale Del Policlinico 155, Rome 00161, Italy, Lazio
e-mail: valeria.panebianco@uniroma1.it

V. Gentile et al. (eds.), *Multidisciplinary Management of Prostate Cancer*,
DOI 10.1007/978-3-319-04385-2_6, © Springer International Publishing Switzerland 2014

Computed tomography virtually plays no role in the detection of PC and its role is limited to lymph node and distant metastases. Molecular imaging with positron emission tomography/computed tomography (PET/CT) systems improves the capability in the staging of PC.

Recently, great interest has been shown in multiparametric Magnetic Resonance Imaging (mp-MRI) which combines anatomic T2-weighted (T2W), diffusion-weighted imaging (DWI), dynamic contrast-enhanced (DCE) and MR spectroscopic imaging (MRSI). The combination of anatomic, biologic and functional information offered by mp-MRI promises to make it a successful imaging tool for improving the Se, Spe and accuracy in PC detection.

6.2   Ultrasonography

6.2.1   Conventional Transrectal Ultrasound

The widespread availability and relatively low costs made TRUS the most widely used clinical imaging method of the prostate. It is mainly used to estimate prostate volume and biopsy guidance; however, it is generally considered to be insufficient for diagnosing or staging PC. Conventional (grey-scale) TRUS is not a reliable tool in identifying foci of PC because at least the 40 % of PC appear isoechoic to surrounding healthy glandular parenchyma and therefore undetectable, thus justifying the poor Se and accuracy of TRUS in detecting PC [2]. The detection rates for conventional TRUS as an imaging modality are calculated to be around 11–35 % [3]. Another drawback is the high operator dependence of the US-based method in terms of the interpretation and repeatability of the examination. Therefore, conventional TRUS is not employed as a routine modality for targeted prostate biopsy, but rather as guidance for systematic biopsies. Up to now TRUS-guided grey-scale biopsy, sampling 6–12 cores, one to two for each sextant, has been the diagnostic standard for PC for many years. The US images provide excellent guidance to the physician with regard to the gland size and boundaries, but limited information with regard to internal glandular tissue and little or no detail on focal lesions. Because up to 30 % of cancer is missed when performing sextant biopsies, the method has been extended to 45 cores for saturation biopsies [1]. Although taking more cores seems to improve the per patient detection rate of PC, the vastly invasive approach of placing up to 45 needles needs to be carefully taken into account.

6.2.2   Real-Time Elastography

The accuracy and detection rate of TRUS-guided biopsy in detecting PC may be increased by means of RTE. RTE relies on the detection of variance in tissue compliance by manual compression and relaxation and exploits the mechanical properties of cancerous tissue, e.g. elevated stiffness resulting from higher cell and vessel density. In a recent study of 139 patients, superior per core cancer detection rates of targeted RTE biopsy over randomised TRUS-guided biopsy were shown.

More than threefold more cancers were detected by randomised biopsy relative to RTE only, suggesting an additional role of RTE-targeted biopsy rather than as a replacement for the randomised approach [4]. Another study evaluated RTE in a cohort of 109 patients with known PC before prostatectomy [5]. In the whole-mount-correlated setting, Se and Spe values of 75.4 % and 76.6 % were found. Brock et al. [6] in a large cohort assigned 353 patients with clinical suspicion for PC to either grey-scale TRUS-guided or RTE-guided biopsy, maintaining a 10-core systematic biopsy scheme, achieving the outcome that RTE-guided biopsy had a significantly higher cancer detection rate (51.1 % vs. 39.4 %), although the overall Se remained low.

Shear wave elastography is a further development of RTE in which the US probe emits acoustic impulses that generate a defined shear wave that allows for the quantitative evaluation of the tissue. This new technique is deemed to be less operator dependent than conventional sonoelastography approach. Early applications of this method have been applied ex vivo [7] and in vivo in 53 patients [8] in order to characterise PC nodules, and high Se and Spe values were observed. Larger patient cohort studies are needed to investigate the reliability of this new emerging imaging technique.

6.2.3 Contrast-Enhanced Ultrasound

Contrast-enhanced TRUS using intravenously injected microbubble contrast agents has been reported to improve PC detection due to increased tumour vascularity [9]. As tumour is usually associated with a higher blood flow, targeted prostate biopsies may be performed. However, the method is limited by the hypervascularity of benign prostatic hyperplasia and prostatitis, which can lead to false-positive results. In a study with 100 men, Mitterberger et al. [10] compared the cancer detection rate between five contrast-enhanced colour Doppler US targeted biopsy cores with 10 systematic biopsies. The authors found that the detection rate for targeted biopsy cores was significantly higher (16 %) than for systematic biopsies (13 %). In a more recent study by the same group [11], involving 1,776 men scheduled for either first time or repeat biopsy, the detection rate with 5 targeted biopsy cores obtained from hypervascular areas in the peripheral zone (PZ) was significantly higher (26.8 %) compared to ten core systematic biopsies (23.1 %).

A recent study combined CEUS and RTE. In 86 PC patients, RTE detected PC with 49 % Se and 74 % Spe. The combination of RTE and CEUS decreased the false-positive value of RTE alone from 34.9 to 10.3 % and improved the PPV of cancer detection from 65.1 to 89.7 % [12].

6.3   Positron Emission Tomography/Computed Tomography

Despite the many advances that have been made with respect to CT resolution, speed and contrast-enhanced CT scanning protocols, including CT perfusion, no clinical role has been identified in the detection of primary PC as a result of insufficient spatial and contrast resolution for the prostate [13]. The only role of CT is nodal and distant metastases staging of PC [14].

On the contrary, PET/CT may play a role in the early diagnosis of PC, although its main indication is the detection of lymph nodes and skeletal metastases.

The role of Fluorodeoxyglucose (FDG) PET is limited in the initial diagnosis of PC not only because of low FDG uptake within prostate tumour cells, but also because of high levels of excreted FDG in the urine; in fact, FDG is concentrated in the bladder and may mask the primary prostate tumour site or locoregional lymph node metastases. Moreover, FDG is avidly taken up by prostatic tissue in non-malignant conditions such as benign prostatic hypertrophy (BPH) and prostatitis.

[11C]-choline has shown greater promise in the detection of primary PC. [11C]-choline, in fact, is taken up in the pelvis exclusively by prostatic tissue and this property is retained by the neoplastic tissue. A major advantage of this radiotracer is its rapid blood clearance (about 5 min) and rapid uptake within prostate tissue (3–5 min). This allows for early imaging prior to excretion of the radiotracer into the urine. Thus, the pelvis can be viewed before significant excretory activity becomes a potential confounder and the prostate is the only organ to have a significant uptake of the tracer in the pelvic region. Unfortunately, the 20 min half-life of 11C restricts the use of [11C]-choline to centres with an onsite cyclotron. In contrast, the longer half-life of 18F (about 110 min) allows transportation of 18F-fluorocholine to centres without a cyclotron. In addition, the shorter positron range of 18F over 11C produces slightly higher image quality. However, 18F-choline has higher urinary excretion than 11C-choline [15].

The local detection of untreated PC by [11C]-choline PET/CT is reported to have a Se of 55–100 %, a Spe of 43–87 %, and an accuracy of 60–84 % in patient-based analyses [16]. Se is related to lesion size. Martorana et al. [17] demonstrated that Se is 83 % for lesions >5 mm and only 4 % for lesions <5 mm. This is not unexpected since the spatial resolution of clinical PET scanners is about 5 mm. Reduced Spe for PC is related to confounding uptake by high-grade prostatic intraepithelial neoplasia, prostatitis, BPH, urinary excreted activity in the base of the bladder or urethra, and by normal tissues surrounding the prostate gland, mainly pelvic sling musculature and rectum [18].

The local detection of untreated PC by 18F fluorocholine PET/CT is reported to have a Se of 64–100 % and a Spe of 47–90 % in patient-based analyses [16].

6.4   Magnetic Resonance Imaging

6.4.1   Mp-MRI

Traditionally, MRI has been used primarily for the staging of disease in men with biopsy-proven cancer. It has a well-established role in the detection of T3 disease, planning of radiation and surgical therapy. Nowadays, prostate mp-MRI has become an increasingly utilised tool for PC diagnosis, staging and response to therapy.

The mp-MRI examination is generally performed as a combination of T2W, DWI and DCE imaging. Some centres will include MRSI, which can be very useful in adding a metabolic assessment. Mp-MRI with either a 1.5 or 3.0-T magnet and with or without an endorectal coil (ERC) is now the preferred and recommended approach to all men presenting for prostate imaging.

In recent years, it has been shown that prostate MRI at 3 T is feasible with sufficient image quality, even without using an ERC [19]. The recent European consensus does not list the use of an ERC as an essential requirement of mp-MRI [20]. However, ERC increases signal-to-noise ratio, which can be applied to gain higher spatial detail and contrast. Heijmink et al. [21] analysed 46 patients before RP who underwent a 3 T examination with body-array coil (BAC) alone and with both BAC and ERC reaching the results that image quality, localisation and staging performance improved significantly with ERC imaging compared with BAC imaging.

In order to allow systematic standardised interpretation of the contribution of the various components of mp-MRI in the prediction of the presence of significant cancer, a scoring system similar to that employed successfully by breast radiologists (BI-RADS) has been approved for mp-MRI (PI-RADS). In this scoring system, every imaging technique (T2W, DWI, DCE and MRSI) is scored on a five-point scale, with a separate T2W description for the PZ and TZ. Additionally, each lesion is assigned an overall score to predict its clinical significance [22] (Fig. 6.1).

Moreover, currently simultaneous imaging PET/MRI systems have been introduced in the clinical practice. PET/MR imaging provides combined structural, metabolic, and functional imaging information that can potentially affect patient management and outcome. Simultaneous acquisition of mp-MR and PET images with an appropriate radiotracer may be particularly valuable for identifying high-yield candidate biopsy sites that could reduce false-negative initial and repeated biopsies [23, 24].

6.4.1.1 T2-Weighted Imaging

T2W provides superior soft tissue contrast and clear delineation of prostatic zonal anatomy [25]. Most PC are low in T2 signal intensity against a background of high T2 signal intensity of the normal PZ, due to loss of normal glandular morphology with PC. However, low T2 signal intensity within the prostate is not always indicative of PC, as other benign conditions of the prostate, such as prostatitis, BPH, scars, or post-treatment changes (i.e. radiation and hormone ablation), post-biopsy haemorrhage, may have a similar low signal intensity. T2W can also assess whether the tumour is organ confined or extending beyond the prostate capsule. The detection of extracapsular extension (ECE) is quite important for preoperative staging because its presence upstages the patient to T3a stage, and thereby dictates a more aggressive treatment approach. On T2W, ECE usually appears as a direct extension of the tumour into the peri-prostatic fat, but ECE may not be obvious in all conditions; under such circumstances, secondary findings should be sought,

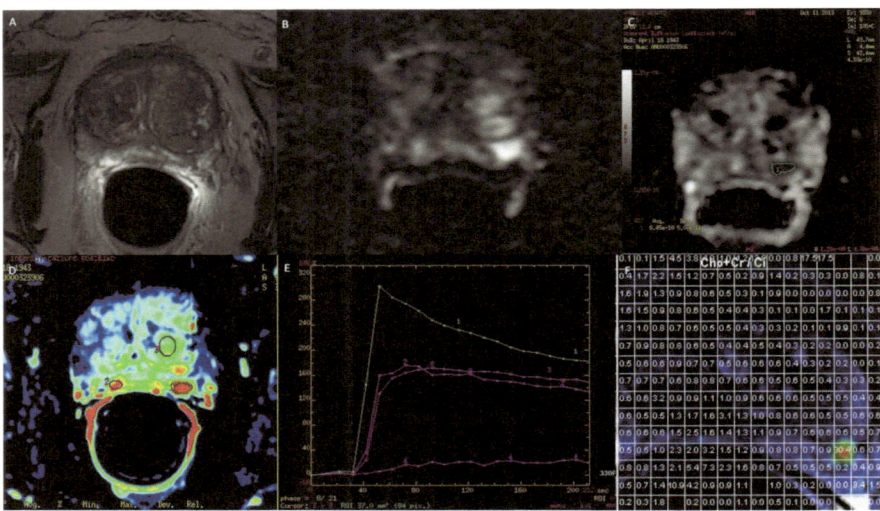

Fig. 6.1 MR images of a 63-year-old patient with prostate-specific antigen (PSA) progression from 3.8 ng/mL (2012) to 4.9 ng/mL (2013). (**a**) High-resolution axial T2-weighted fast spin-echo image showing a focal hypointense zone at the midperipheral gland in the postero-lateral location, without extracapsular extension: score 4. (**b**) Axial DWI image with b-value 3,000 mm²/s and (**c**) ADC map showing restricted diffusion phenomena of water molecules in the hypointense focus: score 5. (**d**) Colour DCE-MR map displaying avid enhancement of the hypointense zone with (**e**) type 3 signal intensity curve: score 4. (**f**) 1H-magnetic resonance spectroscopic imaging reveals in the zone of altered morpho-funcional MRI patterns, a choline-plus-creatine-to-citrate peak integral ratio greater than 1: score 5. The overall score of the lesion is PI-RADS 5: clinically significant cancer is highly likely to be present

including asymmetry of the neurovascular bundle, capsular obscuration or retraction and obliteration of the rectoprostatic angle. Seminal vesicle invasion (SVI) can be seen as a low signal defect within the normally high signal seminal vesicles (Fig. 6.2).

T2W alone is reported to have a wide range of Se and Spe for detecting PC (reported Se: 27–100 %; reported Spe 32–99 %), as well as for staging (reported Se 14–100 %, reported Spe 67–100 %) [26]. A recent study by Kim et al. [27] showed T2W alone at the high field strength (i.e. 3 T) revealing a detection accuracy of 80–90 % for tumour foci larger than 1.0 cm in diameter. However, for smaller tumours, T2W was far less accurate [28]. Concerning the evaluation of ECE, in a cohort of 108 patients, Bloch et al. [29] evaluated the role of T2W and DCE in staging PC and found an overall Se, Spe, PPV and NPV for ECE of 75, 92, 79 and 91 %, respectively. Calculi or clot within the seminal vesicles as well as unilateral atrophy can mimic SVI. However, combined use of T2W with DCE and DWI is helpful in this setting. In addition to lesion detection and local staging, T2W can also provide information about lesion size, which can be important in choosing the best treatment approach.

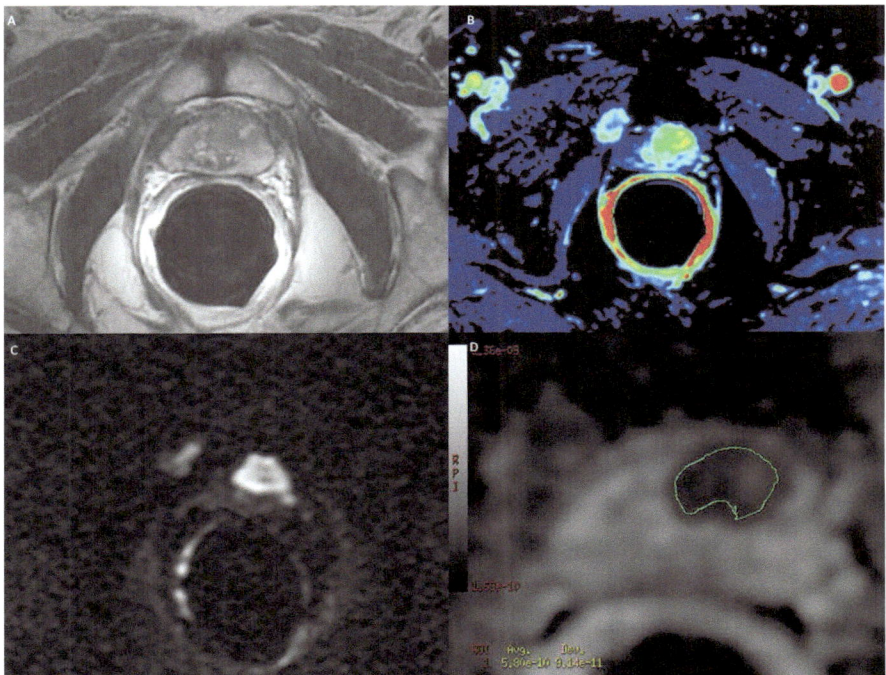

Fig. 6.2 MR images of a 75-year-old man with five negative TRUS-guided biopsies, PSA serum level of 32 ng/mL and PCa3 = 62. (**a**) High-resolution axial T2-weighted fast spin-echo image showing a focal oval-shaped hypointense lesion in the central zone with extension beyond of the anterior capsule. (**b**) Colour DCE-MR map displaying mild enhancement of the hypointense zone with. (**c**) Axial DWI image with b-value 3,000 mm^2/s and (**d**) ADC map showing restricted diffusion phenomena of water molecules in the hypointense focus detected on T2-weighted images. Pathologic correlation after radical prostatectomy yielded central zone tumour

6.4.1.2 Diffusion-Weighted Imaging

DWI is based on an Echo-Planar sequence and depicts the diffusivity of water molecules along the three space directions within the tissue, which is decreased in the densely packed cellular structures of PC. DWI can be used to detect PC due to the lower ADC values of malignant tumours compared with non-cancerous prostate tissue. PCs within the PZ are hyperintense relative to a normal PZ on DWI and hypointense on ADC maps relative to a normal PZ. Recent evidence points to a correlation between a higher Gleason grade and lower diffusivity (low ADC) in PC [30]. Such a finding may, in the future, allow the non-invasive assessment of the histologic cancer grade. In general, at this time, an ADC below 1×10^{-3} mm^2/s is regarded as suspicious for cancer [31]. The addition of DWI to standard imaging protocols dramatically improves the overall diagnostic efficacy of MRI for PC detection [32].

Diffusion tensor technique (DTI) is another Echo-Planar imaging technique that exploits the diffusivity of water molecules to map the orientation of sub-millimetric nerve fibres that unlike DWI highlights the diffusivity of water molecules along several space directions within the tissue. To date, DTI tractography has shown promising results in the visualisation of periprostatic nerve plexus. This information could be useful for guiding proper nerve-sparing surgery using an intra-fascial or extra-fascial robotic approach, thereby ensuring recovery of erectile function after RP [33].

6.4.1.3 Dynamic Contrast-Enhanced Imaging

DCE consists of the acquisition of sequential images using T1-weighted sequences during the passage of a contrast agent (such as low molecular weight gadolinium chelates) within the prostatic tissue. The pharmacokinetics of gadolinium-based contrast agents in the prostate produce different enhancement patterns in PC and benign tissues. The technique is based on the assessment of neoangiogenesis, which is an integral feature of tumours. DCE parameters can often be estimated both qualitatively and quantitatively. The main DCE parameters evaluated are: time to contrast peak (TTP), maximum slope of the contrast enhancement curve (MaxSlope), and area under the contrast enhancement curve (AUC). PC is characterised by a short TTP, high MaxSlope and a high AUC value [34]. However, abnormal enhancement patterns can be seen in BPH nodules and inflammation, making assessment of the central gland difficult [35]. Furthermore, smaller and low-grade tumour foci frequently do not show abnormal enhancement on DCE [36]. For the detection of tumours, DCE alone has a Se and Spe range of 46–96 % and 74–96 %, respectively. A recent work by Puech et al. analysed the performance of DCE in identifying and localising intraprostatic cancer foci in relation to cancer volume at histology. The Se and Spe of DCE for the identification of tumour foci of any volume were 32 and 95 %, respectively. For the identification of tumour foci >0.5 mL, the Se and Spe were 86 and 94 %, respectively, and the AUC was 0.874 [37]. The transitional zone (TZ) is a challenging area for tumour detection, as BPH nodules often show early and intense enhancement, much like tumours. However, similar to tumours in the PZ, TZ tumours also show early washout, which is unusual in BPH nodules. Nonetheless, it is important to interpret DCE of the TZ in the context of the T2W results. BPH nodules can often be distinguished by a clear capsular demarcation and a rounded appearance. It is uncommon for a BPH nodule to contain cancer.

DCE suffers from a relatively lower spatial resolution, so it must be combined with T2W to improve PC detection and local staging (AUC 95 % overall staging accuracy), compared with each technique alone [38]. DCE plays a key role in confirming a suspicion of SVI detected via T2W and/or DWI. The presence of early enhancement within a suspected seminal vesicle lesion strongly suggests invasion. Ogura et al. [39] reported that early, intense enhancement of the seminal vesicles has an accuracy rate of 97 % for SVI.

6.4.1.4 1H Spectroscopic Imaging

MRSI is a functional method used to assess prostate tissue metabolism. Each volume of interest (voxel) acquired in a 3D MRSI contains a metabolite spectra demonstrating the relative concentrations of metabolites such as citrate (Ci), creatine (Cr) and choline (Cho). PCs are characterised by increased levels of Cho and decreased levels of Ci, whereas normal prostate tissues contain high levels of Ci and relatively low levels of Cho and Cr. Thus, the increasing in the Cho + Cr/Ci and Cho/Ci are a marker for PC. Unfortunately, some benign conditions, such as prostatitis and postbiopsy changes, may also result in an increase of the ratio [40].

MRSI has been studied for several decades, and its joint use with T2W has been shown to aid in tumour volume estimation and tumour localisation. However, a recent prospective multicentre study carried out by the American College of Radiology Imaging Network to determine the benefit of combined ERC MRI and MRSI concluded that T2W alone and combined T2W-MRSI had similar accuracy in PZ cancer localisation (AUC, 0.60 vs. 0.58, respectively; $P > 0.05$) [41]. On the other hand, in a recent study, Selnaes et al. [42] found that combined T2W-MRSI performed better than T2W alone, with AUCs of 0.90 vs. 0.85. A principal advantage of the addition of MRSI to mp-MRI is its specificity [43].

6.4.1.5 Targeted-Biopsy Imaging Guided

Mp-MRI examination shows promising results in identifying suspicious foci of PC suitable for a rebiopsy in patients with persistently elevated PSA level and negative TRUS-guided biopsy.

Panebianco et al. in a prospective randomised trial conducted on 150 patients with initial negative TRUS-guided biopsy found that the combination of MRSI and DCE yielded 93.7 % Se, 90.7 % Spe, 88.2 % PPV, 95.1 % NPV and 90.9 % accuracy in detecting PC [44].

Bussetto et al. in a prospective study assessed the role of mp-MRI and urinary prostate cancer gene 3 (PCA3) test in identifying PC in 171 patients with negative prostate biopsy findings and a persistent high PSA serum level. The Se and Spe of the PCA3 test and mp-MRI was 68 % and 49 % and 74 % and 90 %, respectively, thus concluding that mp-MRI increases the accuracy and Se of the PCA3 test [45]. Sciarra et al. in a cohort population of 180 cases also show that in patients with a previous negative biopsy and persistently elevated PSA levels, the use of mp-MRI for indicating sites suitable for rebiopsy can significantly improve the sensitivity of the PCA3 test in the diagnosis of PC [46].

The data yielded by mp-MRI can be used to plan a transperineal MR-guided biopsy (MRGB). The in-bore approaches are exclusively MR based, using prebiopsy MRI to define the targets and real-time MRI to guide and control, with image confirmation, all steps of the procedure. The out-of-bore approaches use US to guide and control the procedure. The results reached by Penzkofer et al. [47] have shown that to date in-bore MRGB is very reliable and relatively easy, and the targeted approach has high yield with more positive lesions coming from ADC and DCE positive sites.

As in-bore biopsies require MR scanners, and thus valuable device time, they are associated with a higher organisational overhead as a result of the magnetic field hazards. Thus, in-bore MRI-guided prostate biopsy can be both time-consuming and expensive. However, it does offer the only method which can image the target and the biopsy needle within it prior to sampling, and thus the only true image-targeted biopsy. A proposed solution for this dilemma is the "out-of-bore" approach with fusion or registration of pre-procedural prostate MRI data to TRUS-guided biopsies, which combines the detection capabilities of MRI with the comparably easy set-up of TRUS [47]. The most straightforward approach for TRUS/MRI-guided biopsies is cognitive fusion, in which TRUS biopsies are performed knowing the localisation of MRI-suspicious lesions derived from peri-procedural MRI [47]. No specialised equipment is required other than an MRI scanner and a conventional TRUS biopsy device [48]. Despite the fact that cognitive fusion seems to improve biopsy protocols, more sophisticated devices have been developed for MRI/TRUS fusion that use different ways of registering the intraprocedural US coordinates to the MRI coordinates [47]. Pinto et al. [49] studied a group of 101 patients from three different risk categories derived from imaging aspects (low, moderate and high) on a TRUS/MRI system developed by Philips. All patients received 12-core standard systematic and MRI/TRUS fused prostate biopsies in the same setting. Cancer was detected in 27.9 %, 66.7 % and 89.5 % of the cases for the low, intermediate and high-risk groups, respectively. In this setting, MRI/TRUS fusion-guided prostate biopsies detected more cancer per core than the standard 12-core approach (20.6 % vs. 11.7 %). Sonn et al. [50] in a recent study concluded that TRUS/MRI biopsy is three times as likely to yield cancer diagnoses (21 % of performed targeted biopsies vs. 7 % of systematic biopsies), on a per patient basis, many cancers were detected by systematic biopsy alone (84 total positive diagnoses, 38 by both methods, 15 by MRI/TRUS alone and 31 by systematic TRUS-guided biopsy alone). Thus, the combination of systematic and TRUS/MRI-guided biopsy seems to be the key in the detection of more cancers.

6.5   How Can Advanced Imaging (mp-MRI) Change the Management of PC

Currently, the radiologists take substantial advantages from the new high technologies, especially mp-MRI. The benefits of mp-MRI include early detection of PC, the decreasing of unnecessary biopsies, the improving of biopsy accuracy, planning surgery, radiation treatment and focal therapies (such as high-intensity focused US, electroporation, focal brachytherapy and focal laser therapy). Thanks to DTI tractography technique, mp-MRI can identify the PC involvement of submillimetre fibres of periprostatic nerve bundles, thus playing a key role in the treatment planning (nerve sparing RP vs. non-nerve-sparing RP); moreover, displaying the anatomical course of periprostatic nerve fibres it is a reliable tool for guiding proper nerve-sparing surgery, thereby ensuring recovery of erectile function after RP [33] (Fig. 6.3).

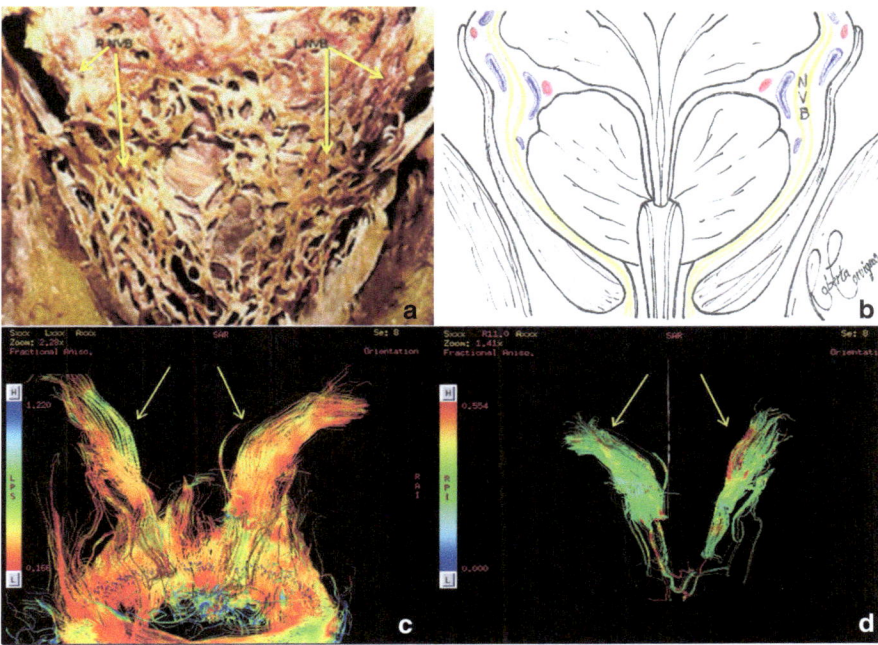

Fig. 6.3 Already published in Eur J Radiol 82(10):1677–82. Coronal view of the prostate. (**a**) The histopathologic corpse section shows the complexity of the neurovascular periprostatic plexus, (**b**) anatomical drawing clarifies the course of the predominant components of NVB. Posterior (**c**) and anterior (**d**) coronal views of a 71-year-old patient candidate for nerve-sparing prostatectomy, obtained from DTI, show the entire nerve plexus (*arrows*), illustrating the irregular fibre courses

An important drawback of mp-MRI is the inability in detecting cancerous foci smaller than 0.5 cc in volume and low-risk Gleason 6 (3 + 3) PCs; these patients, according to EAU guidelines, have the similar characteristic to be included in the active surveillance (AS) (Fig. 6.4). Turkebey et al. [51], in a study with a patient population of 133 patients who underwent mp-MRI at 3.0 T before RP, validated the capability of mp-MRI in identifying patients with PC who would most appropriately be candidates for AS according to current guidelines. They compared the results of mp-MRI with those of conventional clinical assessment scoring systems, including the D'Amico, Epstein and Cancer of the Prostate Risk Assessment (CAPRA) systems, on the basis of findings at prostatectomy. The Se, PPV and overall accuracy, respectively, were 93 %, 25 % and 70 % for the D'Amico system, 64 %, 45 % and 88 % for the Epstein criteria, and 93 %, 20 % and 59 % for the CAPRA scoring system for predicting AS candidates, while mp-MR imaging had a sensitivity of 93 %, a PPV of 57 % and an overall accuracy of 92 %, thus demonstrating how mp-MRI could be considered as a valid tool for non-invasively identifying and monitoring those patients with low-risk PC who traditionally are followed up with regular biopsies.

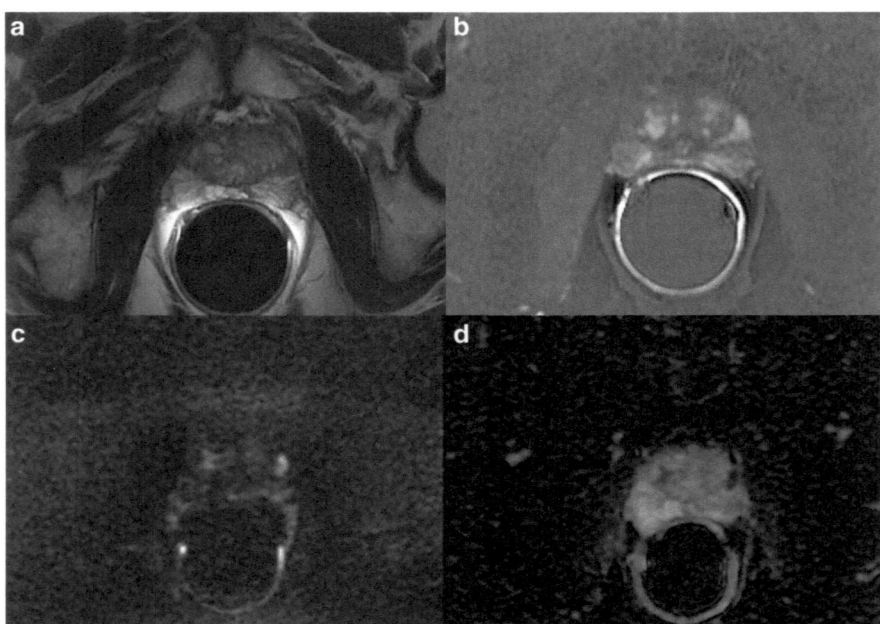

Fig. 6.4 MR images of a 61-year-old man scheduled for active surveillance (AS) [Gleason 6 (3 + 3), PSA serum level of 1.1 ng/mL], who after an mp-MRI examination, underwent a radical retropubic prostatectomy. (**a**) High-resolution axial T2-weighted fast spin-echo image showing a marked hypointense zone at the midperipheral gland in the antero-lateral location, with a mild focal bulging of the prostatic capsule. (**b**) Axial perfusion gradient-echo T1-weighted subtracted image showing avid enhancement of the nodule. (**c**) Axial DWI image with b-value 3,000 mm²/s and (**d**) ADC map showing restricted diffusion phenomena of water molecules in the hypointense focus. Pathologic correlation after radical prostatectomy yielded a Gleason 9 (4 + 5) adenocacinoma

Moreover, mp-MRI could be also considered as a valid tool to push the patients out of AS.

According to ESUR guidelines, the two main clinical indications for an mp-MRI examination are patients with positive TRUS-guided biopsy for the locoregional staging and patients with persistently elevated PSA values and negative biopsy to identify the foci of suspicious PC in order to target a TRUS-guided rebiopsy.

Currently, according to our PC unit within an MDT approach, in a real clinical suspicion of PC—with young age, familiarity, suspicious PSA Velocity and Density in addition to other test as PCA3—mp-MRI is used as the first examination to rule out clinically significant disease (avoiding unnecessary prostate biopsy) and thus to identify those patients who can benefit from AS, to push the patients out of AS and also to target the first time TRUS-guided biopsy.

Conclusions

Currently, given the wide range of available diagnostic techniques and especially the predominant input of mp-MRI in the diagnostic algorithm of PC, the Radiologist can represent a watershed between the different therapeutical approaches. For this reason, our Prostate Unit is composed by two different coordinators: one for the therapy choice—an Urologist—and the other for the diagnostic approach—a Radiologist. The Radiologist uppermost is able to indicate, with the right timing, the best diagnostic technique to use for a given clinical need and then helps the clinician in the subsequent choice of therapy. In a multidisciplinary team approach, the Radiologist can guide the clinicians to send the patient in the right direction based on clinical indication.

Accurate detection and local staging of PC is important for delivering optimal treatment to the patient. Mp-MRI is currently the most accurate technique for the detection of PC non-invasively and is being increasingly used to guide-targeted prostate biopsies. We hope that mp-MRI could be used as first examination in the population with persistently elevated or rising PSA levels to rule out clinically significant disease and thus avoiding unnecessary prostate biopsy to identify those patients who could benefit from AS follow-up or to target the first time TRUS-guided biopsy. Two new approaches to prostate biopsy are under investigation. Both use pre-biopsy MRI to define potential targets for sampling, and the biopsy is performed either with direct real-time MR guidance (in-bore) or MR fusion/registration with TRUS images (out-of-bore). In-bore and out-of-bore MRI-guided prostate biopsies have the advantage of using the MR target definition for the accurate localisation and sampling of targets or suspicious lesions.

References

1. Scattoni V, Raber M, Abdollah F, Roscigno M, Dehò F, Angiolilli D et al (2010) Biopsy schemes with the fewest cores for detecting 95 % of the prostate cancers detected by a 24-core biopsy. Eur Urol 57(1):1–8
2. Ellis WJ, Brawer MK (1994) The significance of isoechoic prostatic carcinoma. J Urol 152 (6 Pt 2):2304–2307
3. Smeenge M, Barentsz J, Cosgrove D, de la Rosette J, de Reijke T, Eggener S et al (2012) Role of transrectal ultrasonography (TRUS) in focal therapy of prostate cancer: report from a Consensus Panel. BJU Int 110(7):942–948
4. Ganzer R, Brandtner A, Wieland WF, Fritsche HM (2012) Prospective blinded comparison of real-time sonoelastography targeted versus randomised biopsy of the prostate in the primary and re-biopsy setting. World J Urol 30(2):219–223
5. Salomon G, Kollerman J, Thederan I, Chun FK, Budaus L, Schlomm T et al (2008) Evaluation of prostate cancer detection with ultrasound real-time elastography: a comparison with step section pathological analysis after radical prostatectomy. Eur Urol 54(6):1354–1362
6. Brock M, von Bodman C, Palisaar RJ, Loppenberg B, Sommerer F, Deix T et al (2012) The impact of real-time elastography guiding a systematic prostate biopsy to improve cancer detection rate: a prospective study of 353 patients. J Urol 187(6):2039–2043
7. Zhai L, Madden J, Foo WC, Mouraviev V, Polascik TJ, Palmeri ML et al (2010) Characterizing stiffness of human prostates using acoustic radiation force. Ultrason Imaging 32(4):201–213

8. Barr RG, Memo R, Schaub CR (2012) Shear wave ultrasound elastography of the prostate: initial results. Ultrasound Q 28(1):13–20
9. Frauscher F, Klauser A, Halpern EJ, Horninger W, Bartsch G (2001) Detection of prostate cancer with a microbubble ultrasound contrast agent. Lancet 357(9271):1849–1850
10. Mitterberger M, Horninger W, Pelzer A, Strasser H, Bartsch G, Moser P et al (2007) A prospective randomized trial comparing contrast-enhanced targeted versus systematic ultrasound guided biopsies: impact on prostate cancer detection. Prostate 67(14):1537–1542
11. Mitterberger MJ, Aigner F, Horninger W, Ulmer H, Cavuto S, Halpern EJ et al (2010) Comparative efficiency of contrast-enhanced colour Doppler ultrasound targeted versus systematic biopsy for prostate cancer detection. Eur Radiol 20(12):2791–2796
12. Brock M, Eggert T, Palisaar RJ, Roghmann F, Braun K, Loppenberg B et al (2013) Multiparametric ultrasound of the prostate: adding contrast enhanced ultrasound to real-time elastography to detect histopathologically confirmed cancer. J Urol 189(1):93–98
13. Ives EP, Burke MA, Edmonds PR, Gomella LG, Halpern EJ (2005) Quantitative computed tomography perfusion of prostate cancer: correlation with whole-mount pathology. Clin Prostate Cancer 4(2):109–112
14. Hovels AM, Heesakkers RA, Adang EM, Jager GJ, Strum S, Hoogeveen YL et al (2008) The diagnostic accuracy of CT and MRI in the staging of pelvic lymph nodes in patients with prostate cancer: a meta-analysis. Clin Radiol 63(4):387–395
15. Hara T, Kosaka N, Kishi H (2002) Development of (18)F fluoroethylcholine for cancer imaging with PET: synthesis, biochemistry, and prostate cancer imaging. J Nucl Med 43:187–199
16. Murphy MA, Kitajima K, Robert C (2013) Choline PET/CT for imaging prostate cancer: an update. Ann Nucl Med 27:581–591
17. Martorana G, Sciavina R, Corti B, Farsad M, Salizzoni E, Brunocilla E et al (2006) 11C-choline positron emission tomography/computerized tomography for tumor localization of primary prostate cancer in comparison with 12-core biopsy. J Urol 176:954–960
18. Murphy RC, Kawashima A, Peller PJ (2011) The utility of 11C-choline PET/CT for imaging prostate cancer: a pictorial guide. AJR 196:1390–1398
19. Scheenen TW, Heijmink SW, Roell SA, Hulsbergen-Van de Kaa CA, Knipscheer BC, Witjes JA et al (2007) Three dimensional proton MR spectroscopy of human prostate at 3 T without endorectal coil: feasibility. Radiology 245(2):507–516
20. Dickinson L, Ahmed HU, Allen C, Barentsz JO, Carey B, Futterer JJ et al (2011) Magnetic resonance imaging for the detection, localisation, and characterisation of prostate cancer: recommendations from a European consensus meeting. Eur Urol 59(4):477–494
21. Heijmink SW, Futterer JJ, Hambrock T, Takahashi S, Scheenen TW, Huisman HJ et al (2007) Prostate cancer: body-array versus endorectal coil MR imaging at 3 T – comparison of image quality, localization, and staging performance. Radiology 244(1):184–195
22. Barentsz JO, Richenberg J, Clements R et al (2012) ESUR prostate MR guidelines 2012. Eur Radiol 22(4):746–757
23. Panebianco V, Giove F, Barchetti F, Podo F, Passariello R (2013) High-field PET/MRI and MRS: potential clinical and research applications. Clin Transl Imaging 1:17–29
24. Hossein J (2013) Molecular imaging of prostate cancer with PET. J Nucl Med 54(10):1685–1688
25. Ravizzini G, Turkbey B, Kurdziel K, Choyke PL (2009) New horizons in prostate cancer imaging. Eur J Radiol 70:212–226
26. Turkbey B, Mena E, Aras O, Garvey B, Grant K, Choyke PL (2013) Functional and molecular imaging: applications for diagnosis and staging of localised prostate cancer. Clin Oncol 25:451–460
27. Kim CK, Park BK, Kim B (2006) Localization of prostate cancer using 3 T MRI: comparison of T2-weighted and dynamic contrast-enhanced imaging. J Comput Assist Tomogr 30:7–11
28. Nakashima J, Tanimoto A, Imai Y et al (2004) Endorectal MRI for prediction of tumor site, tumor size, and local extension of prostate cancer. Urology 64:101–105

29. Bloch BN, Genega EM, Costa DN et al (2012) Prediction of prostate cancer extracapsular extension with high spatial resolution dynamic contrast-enhanced 3-T MRI. Eur Radiol 22:2201–2210
30. Hambrock T, Somford DM, Huisman HJ, van Oort IM, Witjes JA, Hulsbergen-van de Kaa CA et al (2011) Relationship between apparent diffusion coefficients at 3.0-T MR imaging and Gleason grade in peripheral zone prostate cancer. Radiology 259(2):453–461
31. Kobus T, Vos PC, Hambrock T, De Rooij M, Hulsbergen-Van de Kaa CA, Barentsz JO et al (2012) Prostate cancer aggressiveness: in vivo assessment of MR spectroscopy and diffusion-weighted imaging at 3 T. Radiology 265(2):457–467
32. Rinaldi D, Fiocchi F, Ligabue G et al (2012) Role of diffusion-weighted magnetic resonance imaging in prostate cancer evaluation. Radiol Med 117:1429–1440
33. Panebianco V, Barchetti F, Sciarra A, Marcantonio A, Zini C, Salciccia S et al (2013) In vivo 3D neuroanatomical evaluation of periprostatic nerve plexus with 3 T-MR diffusion tensor imaging. Eur J Radiol 82(10):1677–1682
34. Sciarra A, Barentsz J, Bjartell A, Eastham J, Hricak H, Panebianco V et al (2011) Advances in magnetic resonance imaging: how they are changing the management of prostate cancer. Eur Urol 59:962–977
35. Concato J, Jain D, Li WW et al (2007) Molecular markers and mortality in prostate cancer. BJU Int 100:1259–1263
36. Noworolski SM, Vigneron DB, Chen AP, Kurhanewicz J (2008) Dynamic contrast-enhanced MRI and MR diffusion imaging to distinguish between glandular and stromal prostatic tissues. Magn Reson Imaging 26:1071–1080
37. Puech P, Potiron E, Lemaitre L et al (2009) Dynamic contrast-enhanced magnetic resonance imaging evaluation of intraprostatic prostate cancer: correlation with radical prostatectomy specimens. Urology 74:1094–1099
38. Bloch BN, Furman-Haran E, Helbich TH et al (2007) Prostate cancer: accurate determination of extracapsular extension with high-spatial resolution dynamic contrast-enhanced and T2-weighted MR imaging e initial results. Radiology 245:176–185
39. Ogura K, Maekawa S, Okubo K et al (2001) Dynamic endorectal magnetic resonance imaging for local staging and detection of neurovascular bundle involvement of prostate cancer: correlation with histopathologic results. Urology 57:721–726
40. Sciarra A, Panebianco V, Salciccia S et al (2011) Modern role of magnetic resonance and spectroscopy in the imaging of prostate cancer. Urol Oncol 1:12–20
41. Weinreb JC, Blume JD, Coakley FV et al (2009) Prostate cancer: sextant localization at MR imaging and MR spectroscopic imaging before prostatectomy e results of ACRIN prospective multi-institutional clinicopathologic study. Radiology 251:122–133
42. Selnaes KM, Heerschap A, Jensen LR et al (2012) Peripheral zone prostate cancer localization by multiparametric magnetic resonance at 3 T: unbiased cancer identification by matching to histopathology. Invest Radiol 47:624–633
43. Turkbey B, Mani H, Shah V et al (2011) Multiparametric 3 T prostate magnetic resonance imaging to detect cancer: histopathological correlation using prostatectomy specimens processed in customized magnetic resonance imaging based molds. J Urol 186:1818–1824
44. Panebianco V, Sciarra A, Ciccariello M, Lisi D, Bernardo S, Cattarino S et al (2010) Role of magnetic resonance spectroscopic imaging ([1H]MRSI) and dynamic contrast-enhanced MRI (DCE-MRI) in identifying prostate cancer foci in patients with negative biopsy and high levels of prostate-specific antigen (PSA). Radiol Med 115:1314–1329
45. Busetto GM, De Berardinis E, Sciarra A, Panebianco V, Giovannone R et al (2013) Prostate cancer gene 3 and multiparametric magnetic resonance can reduce unnecessary biopsies: decision curve analysis to evaluate predictive models. Urology 82(6):1355–1362
46. Sciarra A, Panebianco V, Cattarino S, Busetto GM, De Berardinis E, Ciccariello M et al (2012) Multiparametric magnetic resonance imaging of the prostate can improve the predictive value of the urinary prostate cancer antigen 3 test in patients with elevated prostate-specific antigen levels and a previous negative biopsy. BJU Int 110:1661–1665

47. Penzkofer T, Tempany-Afdhal CM (2013) Prostate cancer detection and diagnosis: the role of MR and its comparison with other diagnostic modalities – a radiologist's perspective. NMR Biomed. doi:10.1002/nbm.3002

48. Moore CM, Robertson NL, Arsanious N, Middleton T, Villers A, Klotz L et al (2013) Image-guided prostate biopsy using magnetic resonance imaging-derived targets: a systematic review. Eur Urol 63(1):125–140

49. Pinto PA, Chung PH, Rastinehad AR, Baccala AA Jr, Kruecker J, Benjamin CJ et al (2011) Magnetic resonance imaging/ultrasound fusion guided prostate biopsy improves cancer detection following transrectal ultrasound biopsy and correlates with multiparametric magnetic resonance imaging. J Urol 186(4):1281–1285

50. Sonn GA, Natarajan S, Margolis DJA, MacAiran M, Lieu P, Huang J et al (2012) Targeted biopsy in the detection of prostate cancer using an office based magnetic resonance ultrasound fusion device. J Urol 189(1):86–91

51. Turkbey B, Mani H, Aras O, Ho J, Hoang A, Ardeshir R et al (2013) Prostate cancer: can multiparametric MR imaging help identify patients who are candidates for active surveillance? Radiology 268(1):144–152

How to Define the Primary Treatment: The Role of Urologist and Radiotherapist in an MDT

7

Stefano Salciccia and Vincenzo Tombolini

7.1 Which Therapy for Localized Prostate Cancer: Considerations in a Multidisciplinary Team

Prostate Cancer (PC) is now represented as one of the most important medical problems facing the male population. In Europe, PC is the most common solid neoplasm, with an incidence rate of 214 cases per 1,000 men, outnumbering lung and colorectal cancer. Furthermore, PC is currently the second most common cause of cancer death in men [1]. In the last 20 years the widespread use of prostate-specific antigen (PSA) as biomarkers for the early diagnosis of PC has led to a stage and grade migration of the disease and it has resulted in the diagnosis of many men with potentially clinically insignificant disease and with localized disease that represented about 90 % of the diseases and for which several curative options are now available including surgery, radiotherapy, and focal therapy [2]. Based on the different treatment options available today, the treatment decision making for patients with localized PC is one of the most challenging medical decisions facing urologists, radiotherapists, and oncologists. Before determining which therapy is most appropriate for a patient, several aspects should be considered and discussed in an multidisciplinary team (MDT): first, in patient with low-risk PC the question is whether *any* therapy is necessary and the role of active surveillance can be considered as reasonable option now. Second, considering surgery and radiotherapy two valid therapies with curative intent and the lack of well-done randomized trials available to guide physicians regarding the superiority of one therapy over another,

S. Salciccia (✉)
Department of Gynecology, Obstetric and Urological Sciences, Policlinico Umberto I, University Sapienza Rome, Viale Del Policlinico 155, Rome 00161, Italy, Lazio
e-mail: stefi_sal77@tiscali.it

V. Tombolini
Department of Radiological, Oncological and Pathological Anatomy Sciences, Policlinico Umberto I, University Sapienza Rome, Viale Del Policlinico 155, Rome 00161, Italy, Lazio
e-mail: vincenzo.tombolini@uniroma1.it

V. Gentile et al. (eds.), *Multidisciplinary Management of Prostate Cancer*,
DOI 10.1007/978-3-319-04385-2_7, © Springer International Publishing Switzerland 2014

Fig. 7.1 Open retropubic
radical prostatectomy:
Incision of the prostatic apex

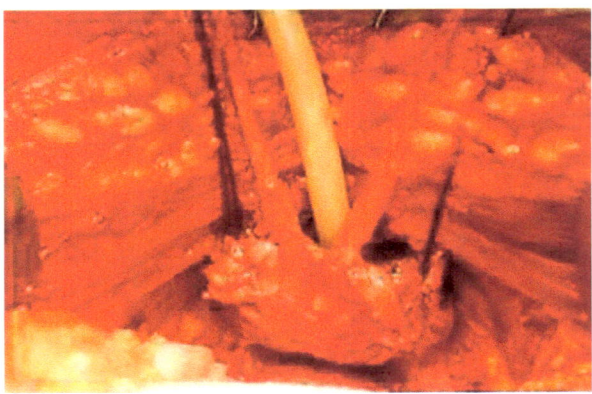

it is important to consider the different side-effect profiles relevant for each
treatment modality. Third, the potential side effects of different therapy impact
quality-of-life outcomes and play an important role for most patients in their
decision making.

7.2   Surgical Treatment: Radical Prostatectomy

The surgical treatment of PC, primarily described by Walsh on 1983 [3], consists of
radical prostatectomy (RP), which involves removal of the entire prostate gland
between the urethra and bladder, and resection of both seminal vesicles, along with
sufficient surrounding tissue to obtain a negative margin (Figs. 7.1 and 7.2). Often,
this procedure is accompanied by bilateral pelvic lymph node dissection. The goal
of RP by any approach (open retropubic, trans-perineal, laparoscopic, robotic
assisted) must be eradication of disease, while preserving continence and whenever
possible potency [4]. Since Walsh first introduced the anatomic nerve-sparing
technique for retropubic radical prostatectomy (RRP), it has become the gold
standard and most widespread treatment for patients with clinically localized
prostate cancer, providing excellent cancer control in most patients with clinically
localized disease [3]. To date there are no studies that have clearly demonstrated
any survival advantage for surgical intervention over nonsurgical therapies among
patients with low-risk prostate cancer [5]. Only one older randomized trial
(106 patients) indicated that radical prostatectomy was more effective in preventing
progression, recurrence, or distant metastases compared with external beam radiotherapy (EBRT) in men with clinical stage T1 or T2 prostate cancer [6]. Overall,
excellent biochemical and survival outcomes can be achieved with any of the
standard used interventions including RP and EBRT, Considering the lack of
well-randomized trial showing a superiority of RP than EBRT, the choice between
two treatments in an MDT should be guided by a careful evaluation of the risks and
benefits for patients on the basis of oncological results and side effects of such
treatment and not secondary by the patient's preferences.

Fig. 7.2 Prostatic bed after removal of the prostate

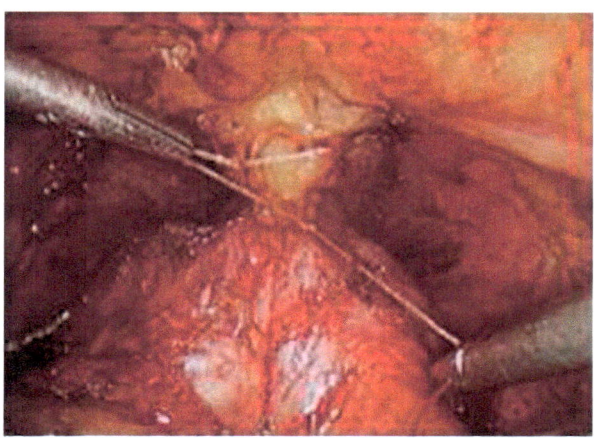

7.3   Radical Prostatectomy: Oncological Results

Today there are several consolidated studies with longtime follow-up showing benefit for RP in terms of overall survival (OS) and cancer-specific survival (CSS), compared with conservative management (Table 7.1). Recently two large randomized trials comparing RP versus observation were published [7, 8]. In the Scandinavian prostate cancer group-4 randomized trial (SPCG-4) 665 patients were enrolled and randomized to surgery or watchful waiting: after 12 years of follow-up, 12.5 % of the surgery group and 17.9 % of the watchful waiting group had died of prostate cancer (difference = 5.4 %, 95 % confidence interval [CI] = 0.2–11.1 %), for a relative risk of 0.65 (95 % CI = 0.45–0.94; $p = 0.03$). At 12 years, 19.3 % of men in the surgery group and 26 % of men in the watchful waiting group had been diagnosed with distant metastases (difference = 6.7 %, 95 % CI = 0.2–13.2 %), for a relative risk of 0.65 (95 % CI = 0.47–0.88; $p = 0.006$). Likewise in the study of Prostate Cancer Intervention versus Observation Trial (PIVOT) [8] after a median follow-up of 10 years, 171 of 364 men (47.0 %) assigned to radical prostatectomy died, as compared with 183 of 367 (49.9 %) assigned to observation (hazard ratio, 0.88; 95 % confidence interval [CI], 0.71–1.08; $p = 0.22$; absolute risk reduction, 2.9 percentage points). Among men assigned to radical prostatectomy, 21 (5.8 %) died from prostate cancer or treatment, as compared with 31 men (8.4 %) assigned to observation (hazard ratio, 0.63; 95 % CI, 0.36–1.09; $p = 0.09$; absolute risk reduction, 2.6 percentage points). After a follow-up of 15 years, the SPCG-4 trial showed that RP was associated with a reduction of all-cause mortality: RR = 0.75 (0.61–0.92). Another interesting data emerges from SPCG-4 study [9]: After a follow-up of 15 years, the SPCG-4 trial showed that RP was associated with a reduction of all-cause mortality, and according to a post hoc statistical subgroup analysis, the number to treat to avert one death was 15 overall and 7 for men younger than 65 years of age. These data suggest that an age > or < of 65 years and

Table 7.1 Studies reporting oncological results after radical prostatectomy for clinically localized prostate cancer

Study	No. of patients	% pT2	% bDFS	% CSS	Surgical approach
Bianco et al. (2005) [4]	1,963	66	82 (5 years)	99	Open
Han et al. (2001) [46]	2,404	51	92 (5 years)	99	Open
Eastham et al. (2008) [19]	1,577	71	91 (5 years)	NA	Open
Ploussard et al. (2010) [47]	911	59	84 (2 years)	NA	LRP
Rassweiler et al. (2006) [48]	5,824	60	91 (5 years)	NA	LRP
Hruza et al. (2012) [49]	500	61	78 (5 years)	98	LRP
Shikanov et al. (2009) [50]	380	87	91 (2 years)	NA	RALP
Patel et al. (2007) [51]	500	78	95 (9.7 months)	NA	RALP

bDFS Biochemical disease free survival, *CSS* Cancer specific survival, *LRP* Laparoscopic radical prostatectomy, *RALP* Robotic assisted laparoscopic prostatectomy

favorable tumor characteristics (PSA < 10 ng/ml and Gleason score <7) could be useful parameters to guide physician in the choice between available treatments. With the intent of reducing the invasiveness of traditional open surgery and improving functional results, several urological centers have developed the technique of laparoscopic RP (LRP) [10]. More recently, Robotic systems have been introduced in an attempt to reduce the difficulty involved in performing complex laparoscopic urologic procedures [11]. The presence of three-dimensional (3D) magnification and tools that are able to duplicate hand movements with high accuracy has allowed many urologists to hypothesize that, despite the absence of tactile feedback, the application of robotic surgery to RP might yield real advantages, not only in terms of shorter learning curves but also in the ability to improve functional results without impairment of early oncologic outcomes. A recent systematic review including studies reporting oncological outcomes for LRP and RALRP had showed favorable results in terms of positive surgical margins rate (PSM): LRP and RALP were associated with PSM similar to those of open RRP [12].

7.4 Radical Prostatectomy in Locally Advanced Prostate Cancer

The incidence of locally advanced prostate cancer at the time of diagnosis has decreased because of the advent of serum PSA screening [13]. Despite this stage migration, a small percentage of patients continue to present with symptoms of clinical stage T3 disease (cT3). Although most patients undergo EBRT plus hormonal therapy, the optimum treatment for those patients is still under debate. Recent progress in surgical techniques has reduced the complication rates related to surgery, and oncological results in this set of patients are encouraging: cancer-specific survival curves at 5, 10, and 15 years that respectively range from 84 to

98 %, 84 to 91 %, and 76 to 84 % of patients, respectively. The overall survival rates at 5, 10, and 15 years range from 78 to 96 %, 63 to 77 %, and $\geq$50 % of patients, respectively. The biochemical-free survival rate (PSA < 0.2 ng/ml) at 5, 10, and 15 years ranges from 45 to 62 %, 43 to 51 %, and 15 to 49 %, respectively. These results are better than the results obtained with isolated EBRT and are of the same order as results reported after EBRT combined with hormonal therapy [14, 15]. RP is a reasonable first step in selected patients with very-high-risk PC and low tumor volume. Management decisions should be made after all treatments have been discussed by a MDT (including urologists, radiation oncologists, medical oncologists, and radiologists), and after the balance of benefits and side effects of each therapy modality has been considered by the patients with regard to their own individual circumstances. The problem remains the selection of patients before surgery. Actually the diagnosis of cT3 diseases is mainly based on digital rectal examination and PSA values [16]; however, Nomograms, including PSA level, stage, and Gleason score as well as new imaging tool as a PET-TC for lynphonode involvement or mMRI for local staging, can be useful in predicting the pathological stage of disease [17, 18].

7.5 Radical Prostatectomy: Complications

7.5.1 Erectile Dysfunction

Given that RP is a curative treatment for early prostate cancer with a proven long-term survival benefit [8], optimal outcomes of RP are not limited to cancer control, but also include urinary continence and preservation of erectile function (EF) [19]. Preservation of EF has become a goal in prostate cancer surgery with advances in our understanding of the prostate and cavernous nerve anatomy and with the introduction of nerve-sparing RP by Walsh (NSRP) [3] (Fig. 7.3). Recovery of EF after treatment for PC has become a main goal over oncological results even more in recent years where the diagnosis is made in younger patients and where different treatments with comparable oncological outcomes are now available. The introduction of NSRP technique has significantly improved the functional results in terms of recovery of sexual function [20] and several studies comparing open RP versus LRP and RALRP have demonstrated a significant advantage for robotic and laparoscopic techniques in terms of recovery of erectile function with a more evident advantage for RALRP [21, 22]. Given that NS technique and the number of neuro-vascular bundles (NVB) preserved are best predictor of recovery EF after RP, there are several preoperative factors that should be considered when physician with the patient faces the problem of what we can expect from surgery over oncological results. A recent systematic review of prognostic indicators for successful sexual outcome showed that the most important preoperative prognostic factors for the return of potency after surgery are the age of the patient and sexual function before the operation: potency rates vary between 61 and 100 %, postoperatively. For men between 50 and 70 years of age the overall potency rate declined to

Fig. 7.3 Bilateral neurovascular bundles preservation
after open radical retropubic
prostatectomy

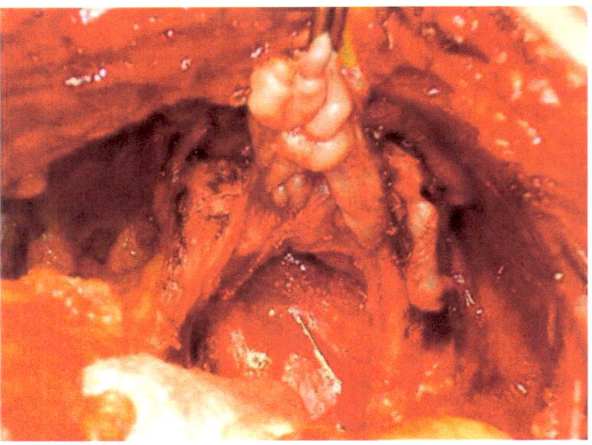

70–85 %. After unilateral and bilateral nerve-sparing procedures potency is found
in 47–58 % and 44–90 %, respectively. Men older than 70 years have low potency
rates ranging from 0 and 51 %, despite nerve-sparing procedures [23]. Based on
these results we can assume that Recovery of sexual potency has become a realistic
option for relatively young patients suffering from an organ-confined prostatic
carcinoma who used to have a normal sexual function before the operation
(Table 7.2).

7.6   Which Therapy for Which Patient: The Point of View of the Urologist

When evaluating a patient with early-stage prostate cancer, the decision regarding
the "optimal" management strategy is complex. It is increasingly apparent that with
the advent of PSA screening, stage migration has resulted in the diagnosis of many
men with potentially clinically insignificant disease [24]. To date there are no
studies that have clearly demonstrated any survival advantage for surgical intervention over nonsurgical therapies among patients with favorable-risk prostate
cancer. Overall, excellent biochemical and survival outcomes can be achieved
with any of the commonly used interventions including RP and EBRT. On the
basis of these considerations, it is important to consider the different side-effect
profiles relevant for each treatment modality and what we can aspect from surgery
in terms of functional results and related quality of life. Today, the best candidates
for RP are those patients with clinically organ-confined disease with comorbidities
that allow a safe surgical procedure. From an oncological point of view, young
patients (<65 years) can expect a significant advantage from surgery in terms of
disease-free survival free (DFS) and it should be considered in a decision-making
process even more in an MDT where urologist, radiotherapist and oncologists
discuss each case suitable for treatment with curative intent. From the point of

Table 7.2 Studies reporting erectile function recovery after nerve sparing radical prostatectomy for clinically localized prostate cancer

Study	No. of patients	Potency definition	Potency recovery % (Mo)	Surgical approach
Kundu et al. (2004) [52]	1,834	ESI	78 (18)	Open
Noldus et al. (2002) [53]	68	ESI	35 (12)	Open
Rogers et al. (2006) [54]	127	ESI	41 (12)	LRP
Hoznek et al. (2001) [55]	134	ESI	56 (12)	LRP
Goeman et al. (2006) [56]	550	ESI	42 (12)	LRP
Curto et al. (2006) [57]	677	ESI	58 (12)	LRP
Menon et al. (2007) [58]	2,652	ESI	70 (12)	RALP
Joseph et al. (2006) [59]	325	ESI	80 (12)	RALP
Patel et al. (2007) [51]	500	ESI	78 (12)	RALP

ESI Erection sufficient for intercourse, *LRP* Laparoscopic radical prostatectomy, *RALP* Robotic assisted laparoscopic prostatectomy, *Mo* Months end point

view of quality of life, to obtain best results from RRP in terms of recovery of erectile function, the best candidate to surgery seems to be a young man with clinically localized disease, with good preoperative erectile function and without comorbidities such hypertension or diabetes.

7.6.1 Radiation Therapy

Primary local management of prostate cancer remains controversial due to the various treatment possibilities available. Traditionally, the primary treatment modalities for patients with clinically localized prostate cancer have included surgical therapy and radiation therapy (RT). Nowadays, it is important to realize the necessity of an MDT for patients with low- (cT1-2a disease, Gleason score ≤ 6 and PSA < 10 ng/ml), intermediate- (cT2b-c and/or Gleason score 7 and/or PSA 1,020 ng/ml), or high-risk (cT3a and/or Gleason score > 7 or PSA > 20 ng/ml). Whereas radiation therapy is recommended as primary treatment modality in locally advanced prostate cancer, because it is improbable to completely excise the tumor by surgery [25], there is no a clear indication for primary treatment in clinically localized disease. There are no modern conclusive randomized clinical trials that compare surgical and radiotherapeutic treatments, and, consequently, there are no data showing superiority of one treatment approach over other [26]. Therefore, the MDT has become a must on the management decision to establish a personal patient's best care therapy. During the decision-making process, patients should be actively involved in the choice of treatment and must be informed of the benefit and risks in quality of life and sexual function of each option, to balanced information [27].

This chapter provides highlights of the curative treatment options, both surgical approach or radiotherapy management. We review the various form of radiation therapy—three-dimensional conformal radiation therapy (3D-CRT), intensity-modulated radiation therapy (IMRT), image-guide radiation therapy (IGRT), brachytherapy, proton therapy—and its outcomes. Regardless of RT form or technique, definitive RT represents a valid treatment option in all patients with localized prostate cancer and it is recommended in locally advanced disease.

7.6.2 Radiation Therapy

Radiation therapy (RT) is continuing to evolve in recent era. Nowadays, the radiotherapy state of the art guarantees different radiotherapeutic approach available to the management of prostate cancer. Over the past 20 years, EBRT has gradually developed and has been replaced by more sophisticated forms of EBRT, such as IMRT, IGRT and proton therapy. These advances in therapeutic methods have turned into a better clinical outcome. Randomized trials have demonstrated that an increase in radiation total dose can safely be achieved without an increase in serious acute or late morbidity, when a highly conformal radiation technique— included three-dimensional photon and proton beams—is used [28, 29]. The significant improvement in radiation therapy techniques has entailed a rise in the cost and in the treatment time. To reduce cost and to increase therapeutic benefit, hypofractionated regime (higher dose per fraction with a shortened overall treatment time) has been suggested as solution, based on the presumed low α/β ratio of prostate cancer compared with surrounding normal tissue [30]. But the real effectiveness of this approach is still uncertain. Likewise, brachytherapy (permanent interstitial implantation, low-dose rate, or high-dose rate) has significantly developed in techniques, optimization, and dose distributions, becoming a valid alternative treatment in early prostate cancer and a co-adjuvant option in selected advanced stage.

7.7 External Beam Radiation Therapy

EBRT represents a well-established primary treatment options for clinically localized prostate cancer, considering that both modern RT and surgery resulted in equal cancer control.

In the last several decades, 3D-CRT has successfully replaced two-dimensional planning treatment, due to significant reduction in grade 3 or greater acute and late toxicity, and implementation of radiation total dose over 70 Gy [31]. Nowadays, the increasing availability of highly conformal irradiation techniques and advances in imaging technology, particularly RMN, are similarly affording new opportunities to optimize RT and diminish toxicity. The primary goal is to increase the dose gradient between target volume and surrounding areas, providing adequate coverage of the prostate and dose restriction to bladder and rectum. With the advent of IMRT, dose conformation and dose escalation have become possible. Of sure, benefit from IMRT requires meticulous delineation of target volume and organs at risk, accurate quality control in radiation planning and delivery, and limiting of

Table 7.3 Studies reporting oncological results after external beam radiation therapy (EBRT) for clinically localized prostate cancer

Study	No. of patients	Dose (Gy)	% bDFS
Kuban et al. (2008) [29]	237	78 Gy	85 (5 years)
		70 Gy	78 (5 years)
Zelefsky et al. (2006) [60]	526	81 Gy	85 (8 years-Low Risk)
			76 (8 years-Intermediate Risk)
			72 (8 years-High Risk)
Thames et al. (2006) [61]	800	70–76 Gy	87 (8 years-Low Risk)
			60 (8 years-Intermediate Risk)
			19 (8 years-High Risk)
Zietman et al. (2006) [62]	392	70.2 Gy	61 (5 years)
		79.2 Gy	80 (5 years)
Zelefsky et al. (2001) [63]	1,100	64.6–86.4 Gy	85 (8 years-Low Risk)
			58 (8 years-Intermediate Risk)
			38 (8 years-High Risk)
Peeters et al. (2006) [64]	664	68 Gy	54 (5 years)
		78 Gy	64 (5 years)
Zietman et al. (2010) [28]	393	70.2 Gy	81 (5 years)
		79.2 Gy	86 (5 years)

bDFS Biochemical disease free survival

interfraction and intrafraction variability—variability that can be reduce and minimize by daily prostate localization using IGRT [32].

EBRT Results The role of radiation dose escalation is essential in tumor control, as supported by the growing evidence from clinical trials. Kuban et al. [29] randomized 301 patients with stage T1b to T3 prostate cancer to either 70 Gy or 78 Gy. The modest escalation dose improved freedom from biochemical and clinical progression (78 % vs. 59 %, $p = 0.004$), with the largest benefit in prostate cancer patients with PSA >10 ng/ml (78 % vs. 39 %, $p = 0.001$). In the Dutch trial [33] patients were randomly assigned to receive 68 Gy or 78 Gy and results showed better outcome in 78 Gy arm (54 % vs. 47 %, $p = 0.04$). In the MRC trial [34] patients were randomized to 64 Gy or 74 Gy and benefited from dose escalation (HR 0.67, 95 % CI 0.53–0.85, $p = 0.0007$) (Table 7.3).

Accordingly, a dose more than 70 Gy is strongly recommended for the treatment of prostate cancer.

Considering the benefit from dose escalation, the debate over treat pelvic lymph nodes versus no treat pelvic lymph nodes still remains, because trials were unable to answer in a definitive way. Pelvic irradiation, with a boost to the prostate, plus neoadjuvant-concomitant-adjuvant long-term androgen deprivation should be considered the standard treatment in high risk and locally advanced non-metastatic prostate cancer; a short-course androgen deprivation may be considered in intermediate risk patients [35, 36] whereas for patients with low risk hormonal therapy should not be used [37].

Table 7.4 Studies reporting erectile dysfunction (ED) after external beam radiation therapy (EBRT) for clinically localized prostate cancer

Authors	No. of patients	Patients potent prior to EBRT n(%)	Follow-up (mean)	ED n(%)
Pilepich et al. (1995) [65]	230	102 (44)	54 months	72 (74/102)
Zelefsky et al. (1999) [66]	743	544 (73)	42 months	39 (211/544)
Hamilton et al. (2001) [67]	457	251 (55)	NA	58 at 12 months 68 at 24 months
Mameghan et al. (1991) [68]	218	42 (19)	NA	45 (19/42) at 24 months
Mantz et al. (1997) [69]	114	NA	18 months	8 at 12 months 25 at 24 months
Turner et al. (1999) [70]	290	182 (63)	23 months	38 (56/146) at 12 months
Nguyen et al. (1998) [71]	101	81 (80)	24 months	49 (40/81)
Beckendorf et al. (1996) [72]	67	40 (60)	NA	33 (13/40)

NA Not available

EBRT Toxicity Gastrointestinal (GI), genitourinary (GU), and sexual complications are the major toxicities that occur during and after EBRT. It is important to pay close attention to dose–volume constraints, because toxicity and its severity are volume related. Patients receiving pelvic irradiation are more at risk than patients treated only to the prostate. Zelefsky et al. demonstrated that using IMRT, acute and late toxicity is significantly reduced compared with conventional 3D-CRT (13 % to 5 %, $p < 0.001$), despite the application of higher radiation doses to the target volume [38, 39]. Acute symptoms develop during the course of RT and resolve 2–4 weeks after treatment. Acute GU toxicity is more common than GI symptoms. Acute GU complications are characterized by urinary frequency, urinary urgency, dysuria, and decreased force of stream, whereas GI toxicity results in enteritis, mainly. The presence of acute symptoms had a significant influence on the long-term devolvement of late toxicity. GU late sequelae are manifest as chronic frequency and urgency; hematuria or urinary incontinence requiring protective padding is more uncommon. GI long-term toxicity, usually, is manifest as proctitis, diarrhea, rectal bleeding, and mucous discharge.

Sexual complications are difficult to evaluate, due to the unclear erectile dysfunction pathogenesis, the patients' comorbidities (such as diabetes or atherosclerosis), and the insufficient quality-of-life studies (Table 7.4); however, it appears that potency progressively decreases 1–2 years after RT, but 50–70 % of patients preserve erectile ability after RT [40]. Considering a period of 10–15 years to be manifest, the very low risk of a second malignant tumor should be taken into account in younger patients.

EBRT Advantage RT has several possible advantages over surgical approach: it should be indicated in all patients, irrespective of age; it is not related to general anesthesia risk; it may have favorable acute GU and GI toxicity profile and assures a good chance to preserve sexual function.

EBRT Disadvantage RT requires a daily hospital presence for at least 7 weeks of treatment with conventional fractionation; RT is not indicated in patients with previous pelvic irradiation or with active inflammatory rectal disease. Acute GI and GU toxicities could be expected, but a low rate of grade ≥ 2 late toxicities is estimated (10–20 %). The induction of a secondary cancer is possible, especially, rectum and bladder cancer, but the data of literature are controversial and the incidence is likely low.

7.8 Particle Beam Therapy

7.8.1 Brachytherapy

Brachytherapy (BT) involves permanent (low-dose-rate brachytherapy: LDR-BRT) or temporary (high-dose-rate brachytherapy: HDRBT) implantation of a radioactive isotope in the prostate. This technique permits to deliver adequate radiation dose to the cancer, minimizing dose to the surrounding tissues, such as bladder, rectum, and small bowel. The selection of BT as monotherapy or as a supplemental boost depends on clinical stage. BT is indicated for patients with low-risk prostate cancer (T1-2a, PSA ≤ 10 ng/ml and Gleason score ≤ 6) as exclusive treatment modality; whereas for patients with intermediate risk disease it is considered in combination with EBRT.

An appropriate patient selection is extremely important, due to the increased risk, between 5 and 10 %, of urinary retention after BT. The initial International Prostate Symptom Score (IPSS) and the prostate volume must be considered. Ideally patient should not have a history of past transurethral resection of the prostate (TURP) or inflammatory bowel disease, a significant urinary outflow obstruction, or an extended prostate volume. Patients with enlarged prostate or at high initial IPSS should be candidates for EBRT.

BT-related toxicity includes irritative urinary symptoms in the immediate post-implantation period or 4–6 weeks after the procedure; usually GU toxicity resolves in 6 months and rarely occurs in chronic. GI complications persist as proctitis in 1–12 % of patients. Posttreatment erectile dysfunction, evaluated in patients who were potent before BT, is reported in 21 % of patients at 2 years after implantation and increase at 53 % at 5 years [41].

Randomized studies comparing long-term outcomes and quality of life after BT, RT (including hormonal treatment), and prostatectomy are lacking. Using PSA as an efficient and robust indicator of the absence of disease, favorable outcome of each treatment, in low-risk cancer, is equivalent (more than 90 %) [42].

BT Advantage BT has the best chance to preserve sexual function versus EBRT and also versus nerve-sparing RP [43]; the incidence of urinary incontinence is very low. The treatment duration is short with one or three procedures.

BT Disadvantage BT requires hospitalization of 2–5 days and a spinal or, rarely, general anesthesia, but recovery is fast. Exclusive BT is not indicated in patients with high or intermediate risk PC and in patients with active inflammatory rectal disease.

7.8.2 Proton Therapy

Proton beam radiotherapy represents a form of charged particles therapy. Although the energy delivered results in a peak of dose (Bragg peak) with a significant dose reduction to nontarget tissues, proton therapy has comparable biological effects related to photons [44]. In prostate cancer only limited clinical trials have compared protons to photons, and, as Mouw et al. reported [45], it is still unknown if the dosimetric advantages of the proton therapy offer any appreciable clinical improvements over IMRT or brachytherapy. For now, proton beam radiotherapy is not recommended as routine treatment.

References

1. Boyle P, Ferlay J (2005) Cancer incidence and mortality in Europe 2004. Ann Oncol 16(3): 481–488
2. Cooperberg MR, Broering JM, Kantoff PW, Carroll PR (2007) Contemporary trends in low risk prostate cancer: risk assessment and treatment. J Urol 178(3 pt 2):S14–S19
3. Walsh PC, Lepor H, Eggleston JC (1983) Radical prostatectomy with preservation of sexual function: anatomical and pathological considerations. Prostate 4(5):473–485
4. Bianco FJ Jr, Scardino PT, Eastham JA (2005) Radical prostatectomy: long-term cancer control and recovery of sexual and urinary function ("trifecta"). Urology 66(5 Suppl):83–94
5. Wilt TJ, MacDonald R, Rutks I, Shamliyan TA, Taylor BC, Kane RL (2008) Systematic review: comparative effectiveness and harms of treatments for clinically localized prostate cancer. Ann Intern Med 148(6):435–448
6. Paulson DF, Lin GH, Hinshaw W, Stephani S (1982) Radical surgery versus radiotherapy for adenocarcinoma of the prostate. J Urol 128:502–504
7. Bill-Axelson A, Holmberg L, Filén F, Ruutu M, Garmo H, Busch C, Nordling S, Häggman M, Andersson SO, Bratell S, Spångberg A, Palmgren J, Adami HO, Johansson JE (2008) Scandinavian Prostate Cancer Group Study Number 4. Radical prostatectomy versus watchful waiting in localized prostate cancer: the Scandinavian prostate cancer group-4 randomized trial. J Natl Cancer Inst 100(16):1144–1154

8. Wilt TJ, Brawer MK, Jones KM, Barry MJ, Aronson WJ, Fox S, Gingrich JR, Wei JT, Gilhooly P, Grob BM, Nsouli I, Iyer P, Cartagena R, Snider G, Roehrborn C, Sharifi R, Blank W, Pandya P, Andriole GL, Culkin D, Wheeler T, Prostate Cancer Intervention versus Observation Trial (PIVOT) Study Group (2012) Radical prostatectomy versus observation for localized prostate cancer. N Engl J Med 367(3):203–213

9. Bill-Axelson A, Holmberg L, Ruutu M, Garmo H, Stark JR, Busch C, Nordling S, Häggman M, Andersson SO, Bratell S, Spångberg A, Palmgren J, Steineck G, Adami HO, Johansson JE, SPCG-4 Investigators (2011) Radical prostatectomy versus watchful waiting in early prostate cancer. N Engl J Med 364(18):1708–1717

10. Guillonneau B, Cathelineau X, Barret E, Rozet F, Vallancien G (1999) Laparoscopic radical prostatectomy: technical and early oncological assessment of 40 operations. Eur Urol 36: 14–20

11. Tewari A, Peabody J, Sarle R, Balakrishnan G, Hemal A, Shrivastava A, Menon M (2002) Technique of da Vinci robot-assisted anatomic radical prostatectomy. Urology 60(4):569–572

12. Ficarra V, Novara G, Artibani W, Cestari A, Galfano A, Graefen M, Guazzoni G, Guillonneau B, Menon M, Montorsi F, Patel V, Rassweiler J, Van Poppel H (2009) Retropubic, laparoscopic, and robot-assisted radical prostatectomy: a systematic review and cumulative analysis of comparative studies. Eur Urol 55(5):1037–1063

13. Hankey BF, Feuer EJ, Clegg LX et al (1999) Cancer surveillance series: interpreting trends in prostate cancer – part I: evidence of the effects of screening in recent prostate cancer incidence, mortality, and survival rates. J Natl Cancer Inst 91:1017–1024

14. Xylinas E, Daché A, Rouprêt M (2010) Is radical prostatectomy a viable therapeutic option in clinically locally advanced (cT3) prostate cancer? BJU Int 106(11):1596–1600

15. Bolla M, Collette L, Blank L et al (2002) Long term results with immediate androgen suppression and external irradiation in patients with locally advanced prostate cancer (an EORTC study): a phase III randomised trial. Lancet 360:103–106

16. Hsu CY, Joniau S, Oyen R, Roskams T, Van Poppel H (2006) Detection of clinical unilateral T3a prostate cancer by digital rectal examination or transrectal ultrasonography? BJU Int 98:982–985

17. Sciarra A, Barentsz J, Bjartell A, Eastham J, Hricak H, Panebianco V, Witjes JA (2011) Advances in magnetic resonance imaging: how they are changing the management of prostate cancer. Eur Urol 59(6):962–977

18. Touijer K, Scardino PT (2009) Nomograms for staging, prognosis, and predicting treatment outcomes. Cancer 115(13 Suppl):3107–3111

19. Eastham JA, Scardino PT, Kattan MW (2008) Predicting an optimal outcome after radical prostatectomy: the trifecta nomogram. J Urol 179:2207–2210

20. Meuleman EJ, Mulders PF (2003) Erectile function after radical prostatectomy: a review. Eur Urol 43(2):95–101

21. Ficarra V, Novara G, Ahlering TE, Costello A, Eastham JA, Graefen M, Guazzoni G, Menon M, Mottrie A, Patel VR, Van der Poel H, Rosen RC, Tewari AK, Wilson TG, Zattoni F, Montorsi F (2012) Systematic review and meta-analysis of studies reporting potency rates after robot-assisted radical prostatectomy. Eur Urol 62(3):418–430

22. Tal R, Alphs HH, Krebs P, Nelson CJ, Mulhall JP (2009) Erectile function recovery rate after radical prostatectomy: a meta-analysis. J Sex Med 6(9):2538–2546

23. Dubbelman YD, Dohle GR, Schröder FH (2006) Sexual function before and after radical retropubic prostatectomy: a systematic review of prognostic indicators for a successful outcome. Eur Urol 50(4):711–718

24. Kollmeier MA, Zelefsky MJ (2012) How to select the optimal therapy for early-stage prostate cancer. Crit Rev Oncol Hematol 84(Suppl 1):e6–e15

25. NCCN (2013) NCCN Guidelines Version 2.2013 prostate cancer

26. Westover K, Chen MH, Moul J et al (2012) Radical prostatectomy vs radiation therapy and androgen-suppression therapy in high-risk prostate cancer. BJU Int 110(8):1116–1121

27. Gomella LG, Lin J, Hoffman-Censits J et al (2010) Enhancing prostate cancer care through the multidisciplinary clinic approach: a 15-year experience. J Oncol Pract 6(6):e5–e10
28. Zietman AL, Bae K, Slater JD et al (2010) Randomized trial comparing conventional-dose with high-dose conformal radiation therapy in early-stage adenocarcinoma of the prostate: long-term results from proton radiation oncology group/American College of Radiology 95-09. J Clin Oncol 28(7):1106–1111
29. Kuban DA, Tucker SL, Dong L et al (2008) Long-term results of the M.D. Anderson randomized dose-escalation trial for prostate cancer. Int J Radiat Oncol Biol Phys 70(1):67–74
30. Lukka H, Hayter C, Julian JA et al (2005) Randomized trial comparing two fractionation schedules for patients with localized prostate cancer. J Clin Oncol 23(25):6132–6138
31. Michalski JM, Bae K, Roach M et al (2010) Long-term toxicity following 3D conformal radiation therapy for prostate cancer from the RTOG 9406 phase I/II dose escalation study. Int J Radiat Oncol Biol Phys 76(1):14–22
32. Jacobs BL, Zhang Y, Skolarus TA et al (2014) Comparative effectiveness of external-beam radiation approaches for prostate cancer. Eur Urol 65(1):162–168
33. Al-Mamgani A, van Putten WL, Heemsbergen WD et al (2008) Update of Dutch multicenter dose-escalation trial of radiotherapy for localized prostate cancer. Int J Radiat Oncol Biol Phys 72(4):980–988
34. Dearnaley DP, Sydes MR, Graham JD et al (2007) Escalated-dose versus standard-dose conformal radiotherapy in prostate cancer: first results from the MRC RT01 randomised controlled trial. Lancet Oncol 8(6):475–487
35. Roach M 3rd, Bae K, Speight J et al (2008) Short-term neoadjuvant androgen deprivation therapy and external-beam radiotherapy for locally advanced prostate cancer: long-term results of RTOG 8610. J Clin Oncol 26(4):585–591
36. Bolla M, Van Tienhoven G, Warde P et al (2010) External irradiation with or without long-term androgen suppression for prostate cancer with high metastatic risk: 10-year results of an EORTC randomised study. Lancet Oncol 11(11):1066–1073
37. McLeod DG, Iversen P, See WA et al (2006) Bicalutamide 150 mg plus standard care vs. standard care alone for early prostate cancer. BJU Int 97(2):247–254
38. Spratt DE, Pei X, Yamada J et al (2013) Long-term survival and toxicity in patients treated with high-dose intensity modulated radiation therapy for localized prostate cancer. Int J Radiat Oncol Biol Phys 85(3):686–692
39. Zelefsky MJ, Levin EJ, Hunt M et al (2008) Incidence of late rectal and urinary toxicities after three-dimensional conformal radiotherapy and intensity-modulated radiotherapy for localized prostate cancer. Int J Radiat Oncol Biol Phys 70(4):1124–1129
40. Pinkawa M, Gagel B, Piroth MD et al (2009) Erectile dysfunction after external beam radiotherapy for prostate cancer. Eur Urol 55(1):227–234
41. Merrick GS, Butler WM, Wallner KE et al (2004) Permanent interstitial brachytherapy in younger patients with clinically organ-confined prostate cancer. Urology 64(4):754–759
42. Levin WP, Kooy H, Loeffler JS et al (2005) Proton beam therapy. Br J Cancer 93(8):849–854
43. Challapalli A, Jones E, Harvey C, Hellawell GO, Mangar SA (2012) High dose rate prostate brachytherapy: an overview of the rationale, experience and emerging applications in the treatment of prostate cancer. Br J Radiol 85(Spl iss):S18–S27
44. Zelefsky MJ, Wallner KE, Ling CC et al (1999) Comparison of the 5-year outcome and morbidity of three-dimensional conformal radiotherapy versus transperineal permanent iodine-125 implantation for early-stage prostatic cancer. J Clin Oncol 17(2):517–522
45. Mouw KW, Trofimov A, Zietman AL et al (2013) Clinical controversies: proton therapy for prostate cancer. Semin Radiat Oncol 23(2):109–114
46. Han M, Partin AW, Pound CR, Epstein JI, Walsh PC (2001) Long-term biochemical disease-free and cancer-specific survival following anatomic radical retropubic prostatectomy. The 15-year Johns Hopkins experience. Urol Clin North Am 28:555–565
47. Ploussard G, de la Taille A, Xylinas E, Allory Y, Vordos D, Hoznek A, Abbou CC, Salomon L (2011) Prospective evaluation of combined oncological and functional outcomes after

laparoscopic radical prostatectomy: trifecta rate of achieving continence, potency and cancer control at 2 years. BJU Int 107(2):274–279

48. Rassweiler J, Stolzenburg J, Sulser T, Deger S, Zumbé J, Hofmockel G, John H, Janetschek G, Fehr JL, Hatzinger M, Probst M, Rothenberger KH, Poulakis V, Truss M, Popken G, Westphal J, Alles U, Fornara P (2006) Laparoscopic radical prostatectomy – the experience of the German laparoscopic working group. Eur Urol 49:113–119

49. Hruza M, Bermejo JL, Flinspach B, Schulze M, Teber D, Rumpelt HJ, Rassweiler JJ (2013) Long-term oncological outcomes after laparoscopic radical prostatectomy. BJU Int 111 (2):271–280

50. Shikanov SA, Zorn KC, Zagaja GP, Shalhav AL (2009) Trifecta outcomes after robotic-assisted laparoscopic prostatectomy. Urology 74(3):619–623

51. Patel VR, Thaly R, Shah K (2007) Robotic radical prostatectomy: outcomes of 500 cases. BJU Int 99(5):1109–1112

52. Kundu SD, Roehl KA, Eggener SE, Antenor JA, Han M, Catalona WJ (2004) Potency, continence and complications in 3,477 consecutive radical retropubic prostatectomies. J Urol 172:2227–2231

53. Noldus J, Michl U, Graefen M, Haese A, Hammerer P, Huland H (2002) Patient-reported sexual function after nerve-sparing radical retropubic prostatectomy. Eur Urol 42:118–124

54. Rogers CG, Su LM, Link RE, Sullivan W, Wagner A, Pavlovich CP (2006) Age stratified functional outcomes after laparoscopic radical prostatectomy. J Urol 176:2448–2452

55. Hoznek A, Salomon L, Olsson LE, Antiphon P, Saint F, Cicco A, Chopin D, Abbou CC (2001) Laparoscopic radical prostatectomy. The Creteil experience. Eur Urol 40(1):38–45

56. Goeman L, Salomon L, La De Taille A, Vordos D, Hoznek A, Yiou R, Abbou CC (2006) Long-term functional and oncological results after retroperitoneal laparoscopic prostatectomy according to a prospective evaluation of 550 patients. World J Urol 24(3):281–288

57. Curto F, Benijts J, Pansadoro A, Barmoshe S, Hoepffner JL, Mugnier C, Piechaud T, Gaston R (2006) Nerve sparing laparoscopic radical prostatectomy: our technique. Eur Urol 49(2): 344–352

58. Menon M, Shrivastava A, Kaul S, Badani KK, Fumo M, Bhandari M, Peabody JO (2007) Vattikuti Institute prostatectomy: contemporary technique and analysis of results. Eur Urol 51:648–657

59. Joseph JV, Rosenbaum R, Madeb R, Erturk E, Patel HR (2006) Robotic extraperitoneal radical prostatectomy: an alternative approach. J Urol 175:945–950

60. Zelefsky MJ, Chan H, Hunt M, Yamada Y, Shippy AM, Amols H (2006) Long-term outcome of high dose intensity modulated radiation therapy for patients with clinically localized prostate cancer. J Urol 176:1415–1419

61. Thames HD, Kuban DA, DeSilvio ML, Levy LB, Horwitz EM, Kupelian PA, Martinez AA, Michalski JM, Pisansky TM, Sandler HM, Shipley WU, Zelefsky MJ, Zietman AL (2006) Increasing external beam dose for T1-T2 prostate cancer: effect on risk groups. Int J Radiat Oncol Biol Phys 65(4):975–981

62. Zietman AL, DeSilvio ML, Slater JD, Rossi CJ Jr, Miller DW, Adams JA, Shipley WU (2005) Comparison of conventional-dose vs. high-dose conformal radiation therapy in clinically localized adenocarcinoma of the prostate: a randomized controller trial. JAMA 294(10): 1233–1239

63. Zelefsky MJ, Fuks Z, Hunt M, Lee HJ, Lombardi D, Ling CC, Reuter VE, Venkatraman ES, Leibel SA (2001) High dose radiation delivered by intensity modulated conformal radiotherapy improves the outcome of localized prostate cancer. J Urol 166(3):876–881

64. Peeters ST, Heemsbergen WD, Koper PC, van Putten WL, Slot A, Dielwart MF, Bonfrer JM, Incrocci L, Lebesque JV (2006) Dose-response in radiotherapy for localized prostate cancer: results of the Dutch multicenter randomized phase III trial comparing 68 Gy of radiotherapy with 78 Gy. J Clin Oncol 24(13):1990–1996

65. Pilepich MV, Krall JM, al-Sarraf M, John MJ, Doggett RL, Sause WT, Lawton CA, Abrams RA, Rotman M, Rubin P et al (1995) Androgen deprivation with radiation therapy

compared with radiation therapy alone for locally advanced prostatic carcinoma: a randomized comparative trial of the Radiation Therapy Oncology Group. Urology 45(4):616–623

66. Zelefsky MJ, Cowen D, Fuks Z, Shike M, Burman C, Jackson A, Venkatramen ES, Leibel SA (1999) Long term tolerance of high dose three-dimensional conformal radiotherapy in patients with localized prostate carcinoma. Cancer 85(11):2460–2468

67. Hamilton AS, Stanford JL, Gilliland FD, Albertsen PC, Stephenson RA, Hoffman RM, Eley JW, Harlan LC, Potosky AL (2001) Health outcomes after external-beam radiation therapy for clinically localized prostate cancer: results from the Prostate Cancer Outcomes Study. J Clin Oncol 19(9):2517–2526

68. Mameghan H, Fisher R, Watt WH, Meagher MJ, Rosen M, Farnsworth RH, Tynan A, Mameghan J (1991) Results of radiotherapy for localised prostatic carcinoma treated at the Prince of Wales Hospital, Sydney. Med J Aust 154(5):317–326

69. Mantz CA, Song P, Farhangi E, Nautiyal J, Awan A, Ignacio L, Weichselbaum R, Vijayakumar S (1997) Potency probability following conformal megavoltage radiotherapy using conventional doses for localized prostate cancer. Int J Radiat Oncol Biol Phys 37(3): 551–557

70. Turner SL, Adams K, Bull CA, Berry MP (1999) Sexual dysfunction after radical radiation therapy for prostate cancer: a prospective evaluation. Urology 54(1):124–129

71. Nguyen LN, Pollack A, Zagars GK (1998) Late effects after radiotherapy for prostate cancer in a randomized dose-response study: results of a self-assessment questionnaire. Urology 51(6): 991–997

72. Beckendorf V, Hay M, Rozan R, Lagrange JL, N'Guyen T, Giraud B (1996) Changes in sexual function after radiotherapy treatment of prostate cancer. Br J Urol 77(1):118–123

Early Diagnosis of Failure After Primary Treatment: Multiparametric MRI Versus PET-TC

8

Flavio Barchetti, Ferdinando Calabria, Orazio Schillaci, and Valeria Panebianco

8.1 Introduction

Prostate cancer (PC) is the most common tumour type among men and is the second leading cause of cancer-related deaths following lung cancer [1].

Currently, modern surgical techniques for radical retropubic RP can ensure good functional results regarding oncological radicality criteria, but the problem of local recurrence after RP is a nodal point due to its high frequency. Commonly, PSA is a non-specific tumour marker but is important to underline that, after RP, the rise of PSA serum levels suggests the presence of local relapse or distant metastases.

On the other hand, a persistently elevated PSA serum level could be due to residual glandular tissue [2]. Tumour recurrence is usually preceded by the rise of PSA serum level and occurs in 20–50 % of patients after RP during a 10-year follow-up [3]; moreover, the biochemical recurrence often is not associated with clinical or radiological evidence of disease. It is well known that in 16–35 % of cases the patients will receive second-line treatments within 5 years from the initial therapy [4]. Freedland et al. [5] showed that biochemical relapse precedes clinical relapse of a median of 5 years and that the time between the end of the therapy and

F. Barchetti
Department of Radiological Sciences, Oncology and Pathology, University of Rome, Viale Del Policlinico 155, Rome 00161, Italy, Lazio

F. Calabria
Department of Nuclear Medicine, IRCCS Neuromed, University Tor Vergata, Rome, Italy, Via Atinense, 18, Pozzilli (IS), 86077, Italy, Molise

O. Schillaci
Department of Biopathology and Diagnostic Imaging and Department of Nuclear Medicine, IRCCS Neuromed, University Tor Vergata, Rome, Italy, Viale Oxford, 81, 00133, Italy, Lazio

V. Panebianco (✉)
Department of Radiological Sciences, Oncology & Pathology, Sapienza University, Policlinico Umberto I, Viale Del Policlinico 155, Rome 00161, Italy, Lazio
e-mail: valeria.panebianco@uniroma1.it

V. Gentile et al. (eds.), *Multidisciplinary Management of Prostate Cancer*,
DOI 10.1007/978-3-319-04385-2_8, © Springer International Publishing Switzerland 2014

the start of the biochemical recurrence represents a predictive value for cancer-specific survival.

According to EAU-guidelines, treatment failure after RP is defined as a rising PSA level and in particular two consecutive values of PSA > 0.2 ng/ml appear to represent biochemical recurrent cancer [6].

Following these criteria, once that biochemical relapse has been diagnosed, it is essential to discriminate between local relapse and distant metastases in order to plan the best therapeutic approach.

For this reason, the clinicians commonly follow some parameters that can help to differentiate between local and distant relapse. According to EAU-guidelines, there are two specific criteria to theoretically assess the localisation of tumour recurrence: the rise of PSA over 0.2 ng/ml within 6–12 months after RP suggests a high risk of local recurrence, whereas a PSA increase within a shorter period of time suggests distant metastases progression. The second criterion used is PSA doubling time (PSAdt). The PSAdt is the time (in months) it takes for the PSA value to double and is measured by the following formula: $PSAdt = [\log(2) \times t]/[\log(PSA\ delay) - \log(PSA\ early)]$ [7].

Several values of PSAdt have been proposed as cut-off to discriminate between local relapse and distant metastases; for some authors, a PSAdt cut-off value lower than 4 months may be more frequently associated with distant metastases, whereas a median PSAdt >12 months predicts local failure [8]. In other papers, it has been observed that patients with PSA increasing within 12 months after radical treatment or with a PSAdt ≤ 6 months most probably have systemic metastases, although those with delayed biochemical failure (i.e. > 24 months after treatment or with a PSAdt > 12 months) more probably have local relapse [9].

Other information can be obtained from the pathological examination after RP. The TNM staging system of the International Union Against Cancer (UICC) recommends to report not only the location but also the extension of extraprostatic invasion, because extension is related to the risk of recurrence [10]. For that concern the surgical margin status, even if there is insufficient evidence to prove a relationship between the extension of positive surgical margins and the risk of recurrence [11], is considered an independent risk factor for biochemical recurrence, particularly local recurrence.

The way of treatment for PC recurrence after RP remains controversial and different therapeutic options are available; in the absence of metastatic disease, a rising PSA level is interpreted as locally persistent or recurrent disease and salvage radiation treatment could theoretically be the first choice of treatment. However, if distant metastases are diagnosed, radiotherapy on the prostatic fossa would be unnecessary, with higher risk of morbidity for the patient, and the relevant treatment consists with hormone deprivation therapy [12].

For all these reasons, there is a strong need for an imaging technique able to recognise small recurrent lesions and to describe the nature of these (inflammation or scar tissue, healthy residual prostate tissue or persistent neoplastic tissue). These technique should be able to detect residual disease when the PSA is very low (<1 ng/ml), so to early perform the best therapeutic option. Nowadays, several imaging techniques are available, but they all have limitations and often fail to produce reliable results. Transrectal ultrasound (TRUS) has neither good sensitivity nor good specificity in cases of early recurrent cancer [13] and at present TRUS-guided biopsy of the prostate bed is not recommended by EAU-guidelines in patients with PSA increase <1 ng/ml. Scattoni et al. [14] demonstrated that TRUS-guided biopsy to detect local relapse after RP have a limited sensitivity of 25–54 % when the PSA is <1.0 ng/ml.

In the recent years, new technological acquisitions have allowed the development of imaging techniques which combine anatomic, biological and functional information. Multiparametric Magnetic Resonance Imaging (mp-MRI) and Positron Emission Tomography/Computed Tomography (PET/CT) have been proposed as useful tools in the early diagnosis of PC relapse. Both MRI and PET/CT nowadays are able to detect changing in cellular metabolism. MRI with spectroscopy shows the relative concentrations of metabolites in the prostate as choline, citrate and creatine. PET/CT is able to visualise cellular metabolism using different radiotracers: 18F-Fluorodeoxyglucose (18F-FDG), 11C-Methionine, 11C-Acetate and choline (labelled with 11C or 18F). The large amount of literature shows that choline is not only the most analysed radiopharmaceutical, but probably is the most useful for the identification of PC cells [15]. The aim of metabolic imaging should be to have an optimal spatial resolution so to detect very small lesions like local recurrences after RP, particularly in patients with biochemical failure and very low levels of PSA.

For the best of our knowledge, both mp-MRI and PET/CT have yielded promising results in the diagnosis of PC, in particular of local recurrence of PC after primary therapy.

8.2 PET/CT

The PET/CT is a molecular imaging hybrid technique that provides in a single whole body session important information on metabolic and functional characteristics of oncologic diseases, with the PET scanner, fused with anatomic information provided by CT component of the exam. Moreover, fused PET/CT images can be evaluated, by dedicated workstations, in multiparametric modality in axial, sagittal or coronal planes.

Malignant tumours are usually characterised by enhanced glucose metabolism. For this reason, the most useful radiopharmaceutical is the 18F-FDG, an analogue of glucose. Rationale for the use of 18F-FDG is the higher glucose metabolism displayed by malignant cells compared with benign cells.

Since PC is a tumour with malignant biological behaviour but very low glucose metabolism, several radiopharmaceuticals have been proposed to evaluate this disease in PET/CT.

Standing to results in literature, the most promising tracer is choline (Fig. 8.1), labelled with 11C (in those PET centres provided by a cyclotron, due to the rapid decay of the nuclide) or 18F (with a longer half-time decay of 110′).

The accuracy of choline PET/CT in staging and restaging of PC has been assessed by several studies [16].

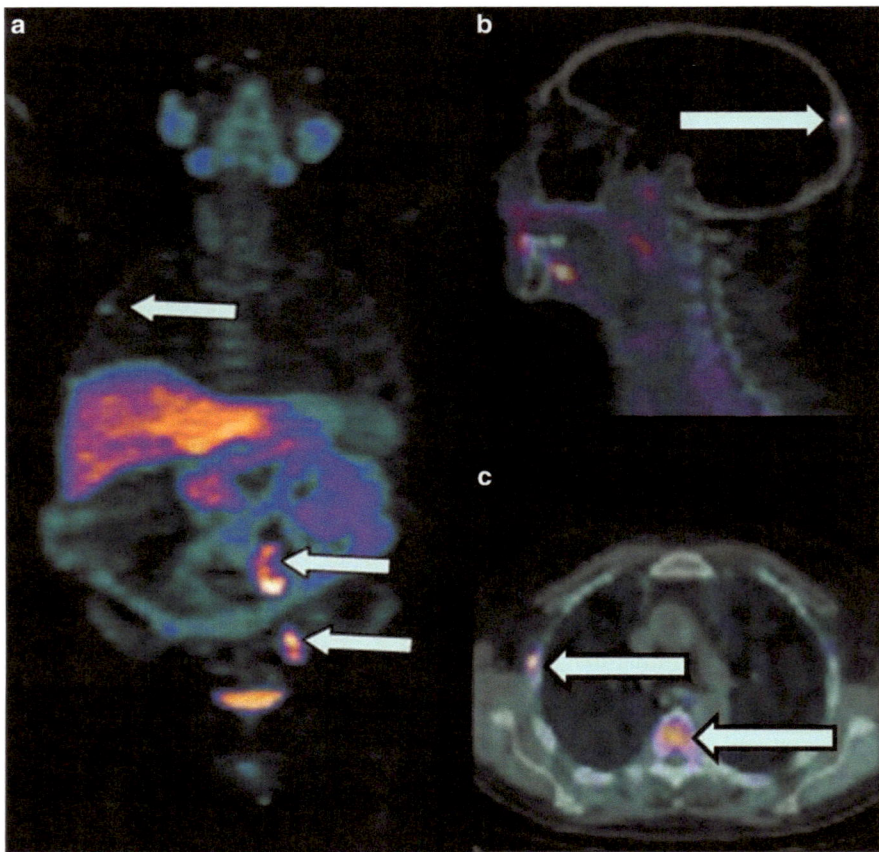

Fig. 8.1 Choline PET/CT images of a 69-year-old patient with biochemical recurrence (PSA serum level 2.3 ng/ml) after radical prostatectomy for prostate cancer. (**a**) Axial coronal fused PET/CT image showing an uptake of the radiotracer at the lateral arch of the III right rib and at the level of left para-aortic and homolateral external iliac lymph nodes. No uptake at the level of the post-prostatectomy bed was found. (**b**) Sagittal fused PET/CT image showing a focal uptake at occipital bone. (**c**) Axial fused PET/CT image displaying the presence of two focal uptake of radiotracer at the soma of T6 and at the lateral arch of the III right rib. All these findings are consistent with bone and lymph nodes metastases

   Choline is a component of phosphatidylcholine, an important element of cell membranes; as known, biosynthesis of the cell membrane is very fast in tumour tissues and the up-regulation of choline kinase activity, particularly increased in PC cells, induces a higher uptake of choline [17].

   This radiopharmaceutical has been employed in detecting various tumours, such as brain lesions [18], lung carcinoma [19] and bladder cancer [20].

   However, its main clinical use is the study of PC, as demonstrated by numerous studies published in recent years. The [11C]-choline, in fact, is taken up in the pelvis exclusively by prostatic tissue and this property is retained by the neoplastic tissue. The [11C]-choline has also a negligible elimination through the urinary tract and the prostate is the only organ to have a significant uptake of the tracer in the pelvic region.

Regarding 18F-FDG, some studies have been showed that PET/CT with choline can detect more metastatic lymph nodes and bony metastatic lesions than 18F-FDG PET/CT in PC patients [21].

Furthermore, Picchio et al. [22] in a study showed that choline PET/CT identified more lesions suspected for neoplastic relapse (42 %) compared to 18F-FDG PET/CT (27 %) and demonstrated that choline PET is more accurate in identifying both local and distant recurrence.

There are several studies on the role of choline PET in the detection of primary tumour in the prostate gland [23, 24] and its use in the staging of prostatic disease before treatment [25, 26], especially in relation to PSA value [27]. However, its role in this field is still not clear, since the uptake of choline can occur in some benignant conditions, such as prostatic hyperplasia or prostatitis.

Therefore, the restaging of PC can be the main field of application of this imaging modality. In particular, the main role of choline PET/CT is represented by its ability to identify the location of the recurrence of the disease in the patients who had already undergone radical surgical treatment for prostate cancer and that present a biochemical relapse [28, 29].

Heinisch et al., in a single-centre retrospective study [30], analysed 31 patients after RP and found that 8/17 patients (47 %) with biochemical recurrence and with PSA <5 ng/ml, had positive results at 18F-choline PET/CT. Furthermore, in this paper, they found malignancy in 7/8 men confirmed by either biopsy or the course of the disease.

Rinnab et al. [31], in a single-centre retrospective study, analysed 50 patients with biochemical recurrence after primary therapy for PC (mean PSA serum levels: 3.62 ng/ml; range 0.5–13.1 ng/ml); the authors considered the sensitivity and specificity of 11C-choline PET/CT only in patients with PSA < 2.5 ng/ml, reporting 91 % and 50 %, respectively. In another single-centre retrospective study, Rinnab et al. [32] enrolled 41 patients with biochemical failure following RP (mean PSA was 2.8 ng/ml; range 0.41–11.6 ng/ml); overall, the sensitivity of 11C-choline PET/CT was 93 %, specificity 36 %, PPV 80 % and NPV 67 %.

Castellucci et al. [33] enrolled 190 patients with biochemical recurrence after RP (mean PSA serum level 4.2 ng/ml; range 0.2–25.4 ng/ml) and found an overall sensitivity of 11C-choline PET/CT of 73 % and specificity of 69 %. The same group [34], in another single-centre retrospective study, analysed 102 patients with biochemical relapse after RP (PSA serum level ranging from 0.2 to 1.5 ng/ml) submitted to 11C-choline PET-CT examination; all suspected local recurrences at PET/CT have been confirmed at TRUS-guided biopsy. Regarding local recurrence, the sensitivity of 11C-choline PET-CT was 53.8 % and specificity was 100 % (no false positive were recorded). Giovacchini et al. [35] in a single-centre retrospective study analysed 170 patients with biochemical failure after RP submitted to 11C-choline PET/CT; the mean PSA serum level at the time of the exam was

3.24 ng/ml (range 0.23–48.6 ng/ml) and mean PSAdt was 9.37 months. PET-CT showed a sensitivity of 87 %, specificity of 89 %, PPV of 87 %, NPV of 89 % and accuracy of 88 %. In this study, PET-CT positive findings were confirmed using histological analysis of lymph node specimen, anastomosis biopsy of the urethra/bladder neck, progression on PET-CT follow-up studies associated with increased PSA level, confirmation with conventional imaging, disappearance or sizable reduction of choline uptake after local or systemic treatment and PSA decrease greater than 50 % after selective irradiation of the unique site of pathological choline uptake.

In a second single-centre retrospective study, Giovacchini et al. [36] enrolled 358 patients with biochemical recurrence after RP: the mean PSA value was 3.77 ng/ml (range 0.23–45.2 ng/ml). 11C-choline PET-CT was performed in all patients and results were validated by histological analysis. Authors reported an overall sensitivity of 85 %, specificity 93 %, PPV 91 %, NPV 87 % and accuracy 89 %.

In the third single-centre retrospective study, Giovacchini et al. [37] from a database of 2,124 patients, retrospectively analysed 109 patients with biochemical recurrence (mean PSA before imaging of 1.31 ng/ml, range 0.22–16.76 ng/ml) who underwent 11C-choline PET/-CT. They reported positive findings at 11C-choline PET-CT in 12/109 patients, as local recurrence in 4 patients and as pelvic nodal metastases in 8 cases.

A relevant limit of all these studies is the lack of information on local recurrence dimensions.

Reske et al. [38], in a single-centre retrospective study, analysed 49 patients who underwent 11C-choline PET-CT examination with mean PSA level 2 ng/ml and median maximal diameter of the lesions of 1.7 cm (range 0.9–3.7 cm); TRUS biopsy was used to validate the results. They concluded that 11C-choline PET-CT had a sensitivity of 73 %, specificity 88 %, PPV 92 %, NPV 61 % and an accuracy of 78 %.

Up to now, the overall choline PET/CT sensitivity in detecting sites of PC relapse ranges between 38 % and 98 %. It has been demonstrated that choline PET/CT technology positive detection rate improves with increasing PSA values.

The most important feature provided by all the cited studies on this topic is linked to the strict relationship between choline PET/CT detection rate and PSA value in restaging PC patients. In the last decade, various authors have been proposed some cut-off values to help in discriminate those patients who can potentially benefit by a choline PET/CT scan; Cimitan et al. [39] proposed that a PSA cut-off value higher than 4 ng/ml is more probably associated to the possibility to detect distant metastases.

It has been found more higher is the value of PSA at the time of the scan, greater is the detection rate of choline PET/CT: 36 % for values of PSA <1 ng/ml; 43 % for PSA values between 1 and 2 ng/ml; 62 % for PSA values of between 2 and 3 ng/ml and 73 % if the PSA ≥3 ng/ml [40].

More recently, several authors proposed lower PSA cut-off values to individuate the patients to undergone choline PET/CT. Rinnab et al. proposed a cut-off value of

1.5 ng/ml but, generally, various authors are in agreement regarding a better sensitivity of the exam when performed in patients with PSA serum level higher or equal to 2 ng/ml [31, 32, 41].

More recently, the attention of the researchers has been focused on the potential role of PSA kinetics such as PSAdt, already cited, and PSA velocity (PSAve), a PSA derivative determined as linear regression of the PSA values over time [9].

In particular, standing to literature data, PSAdt and PSAve values are correlated with specific mortality risk of PC [42]. Additionally, it has been well reported that the risk of distant metastases in patients with biochemical failure after RP depends on PSA and PSAdt values. In particular, it has been showed that when PSAdt is more than 6 months, the risk of metastasis is less than 3 %, even with absolute PSA values of >30 ng/ml. If PSAdt is less than 6 months and PSA is >10 ng/ml, the risk of metastasis is near to 50 % [43].

Partin et al. [44] evaluated the usefulness of PSAve in predicting recurrence after RP and found that combining data relative to PSAve, Gleason score and pathological staging is helpful in distinguishing local recurrence from distant metastases.

Generally, a PSAdt the sensitivity of choline PET/CT is significantly higher in patients with a PSAve >2 ng/ml/year or a PSAdt ≤6 months [45]. In the cited study, in particular, the proposed PSAve cut-off of 2 ng/ml/year seemed to more accurately separate patients with a positive PET/CT scan from those with a negative scan, even if other authors suggest that the patients with a PSAve >1 ng/ml/year should be submitted to choline PET/CT [46].

In all cited studies, the very good detection rate or the sensitivity of choline PET/CT is often associated with distant metastases (for both lymph node and bone metastases) while the data about the diagnosis of local relapse are still discordant. In particular, when the mean PSA level is lower than <1.5 ng/ml, the detection rate of choline PET/CT for local recurrence is definitely poor, probably because of low PET spatial resolution limits (5–6 mm) which do not allow the detection of small lesions.

In a review article, Picchio et al. [41] confirm that the routine use of choline PET/CT for localisation of local relapse of PC cannot be recommended for PSA values <1 ng/ml.

In synthesis, standing to literature data, the choline PET/CT could play a role in management of PC patients, in particular during the restaging, with a good sensitivity regarding distant metastases and good detection rate in relationship to PSA value higher than 2 ng/ml, PSAdt lower than 6 months and PSAve higher than 2 ng/ml/year. To date, its role in detecting local recurrence in prostatic fossa after radical surgical treatment still remains unclear.

8.3   Mp-MRI

In the last 20 years, several progresses have been done in the use of MRI. High-field strength endorectal coil MRI is able to produce a morphological imaging of the prostate, particularly with T2-weighted imaging. Other recent complementary functional techniques that are Dynamic contrast-enhanced MRI (DCE-MRI), 1H-spectroscopic imaging (1H-MRSI) and Diffusion-weighted imaging (DWI) improve the staging and the detection of PC. DCE-MRI is a technique based on Gradient-Echo T1-weighted sequences used during the passage of a gadolinium contrast agent in order to assess the neoangiogenesis; therefore, it can detect those tumours in which an angiogenic pathway has been turned on [47]. DWI yields qualitative and quantitative information about tissue cellularity and cell membrane integrity. Intraductal and extracellular water molecules move freely. In PC, extracellular space is decreased; therefore, the water molecule movement is restricted and the so-called apparent diffusion coefficient values are low. DWI can be produced without the administration of exogenous contrast medium and can be considered the most practical and simple to use [48]. MRSI is a three-dimensional data set of the prostate, with volume elements (voxels) ranging from 0.24 to 0.34 cm [49]. This technique produces the relative concentration of metabolites within voxels, such as citrate, choline and creatine. Recent studies demonstrate that in PC citrate levels are reduced, creatine and particularly choline are elevated. The peak integral ratio of choline plus creatine to citrate can distinguish from PC tissue to healthy tissue [50]. On the basis of the literature, each voxel can be categorised as follows: fibrotic or scar tissue when the ratio is <0.2, residual healthy prostatic glandular tissue when ratio is >0.2 and <0.5, probably recurrent PC when ratio is >0.5 and <1 and definitively recurrent PC tissue when ratio is >1 [51]. MRSI technique is more complex when compared with DWI or DCE-MRI and it also requires longer acquisition times. Mp-MRI has the advantage to have a very good spatial resolution so as to localise and characterise PC, to detect very small lesions and to better differentiate from healthy to neoplastic areas. It is a complex technique and needs experienced and trained radiologists, in particular if MRSI is considered.

Recently, mp-MRI more than other imaging procedures (Figs. 8.2 and 8.3) has been proposed as a useful tool in the diagnosing of local recurrence of PC after RP [52].

Once biochemical progression of PSA serum level has been diagnosed after RP, it is essential for treatment planning to determine whether the recurrence has developed at local or distant sites, but the possibility of residual glandular tissue should be taken into account. In this setting, diagnostic imaging techniques are useful to differentiate local cancer recurrence from systemic relapse and to direct patients to the best therapeutic approach, that is, radiotherapy for local recurrence and hormone therapy for systemic disease [12]. Moreover, it is very important for radiation oncologists to differentiate residual prostatic healthy tissue from local recurrence because the dose of radiation therapy is different [53].

Choline PET/CT is recommended when PSA serum value is higher than 1 ng/ml because this technique has good sensitivity and specificity in detecting lymph nodes, distant recurrence and local recurrences after RP only in patients with high PSA values. Moreover, the ability of choline PET/CT in detecting local recurrence depends on lesion size, being usually higher if the lesion is more than 1 cm in diameter [54].

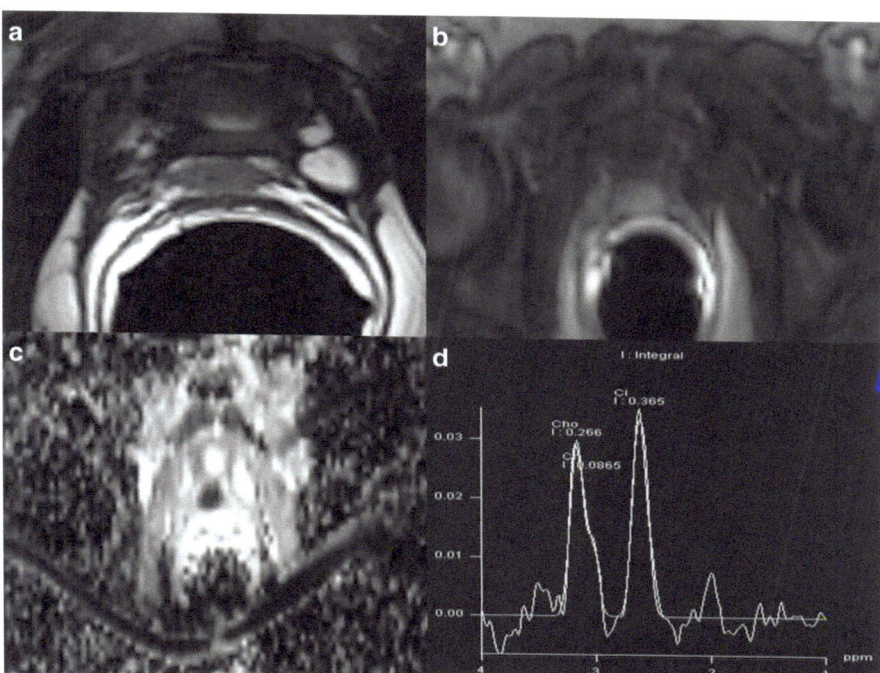

Fig. 8.2 Multiparametric-MR images of a 64-year-old man with prostate-specific antigen progression (PSA serum level 0.75 ng/ml) after radical retropubic prostatectomy, with suspected local recurrence. (**a**) Axial T2-weighted fast spin-echo image shows a solid tissue of 1 cm in size on posterior perianastomotic location in front of the rectal wall at about 40 mm from the ureteral meatus which is slightly hyperintense compared to pelvic muscles. (**b**) Axial Gradient-echo T1-weighted image showing a remarkable enhancement of the pathological tissue. (**c**) Axial ADC map reconstructed from images obtained at *b* values of 0, 500 and 1,000 s/mm shows a dark area corresponding to the abnormal hyperintense tissue seen on T2-weighted images. (**d**) 1H-magnetic resonance spectroscopic imaging reveals a high choline peak with a choline-plus-creatine-to-citrate ratio greater than 0.9. All these findings are consistent with local recurrence

Although Ch-PET/CT is recommended for high PSA values, in patients with low biochemical alterations after RP ($0.2 < PSA < 1$ ng/ml) it is very important for radiation oncologists to exclude the presence of locoregional relapse.

Within mp-MRI, DCE-MRI has proved to be the most reliable technique in depicting locoregional relapse [55–58].

Up to now, there are several studies which demonstrate the usefulness of MRI in detecting local cancer recurrence. At present, mp-MRI after RP is indicated to diagnose small local recurrence and—thanks to functional imaging—to distinguish between residual glandular tissue and or/fibrosis and nodule recurrence; it may also be able to determine the aggressiveness of nodule recurrence. Panebianco et al. [59] compared ADC values of local recurrences with the histological results. The mean and standard deviation of ADC values were 0.5 ± 0.23 mm^2/s for high-grade aggressiveness recurrence, 0.8 ± 0.09 mm^2/s for intermediate-grade aggressiveness

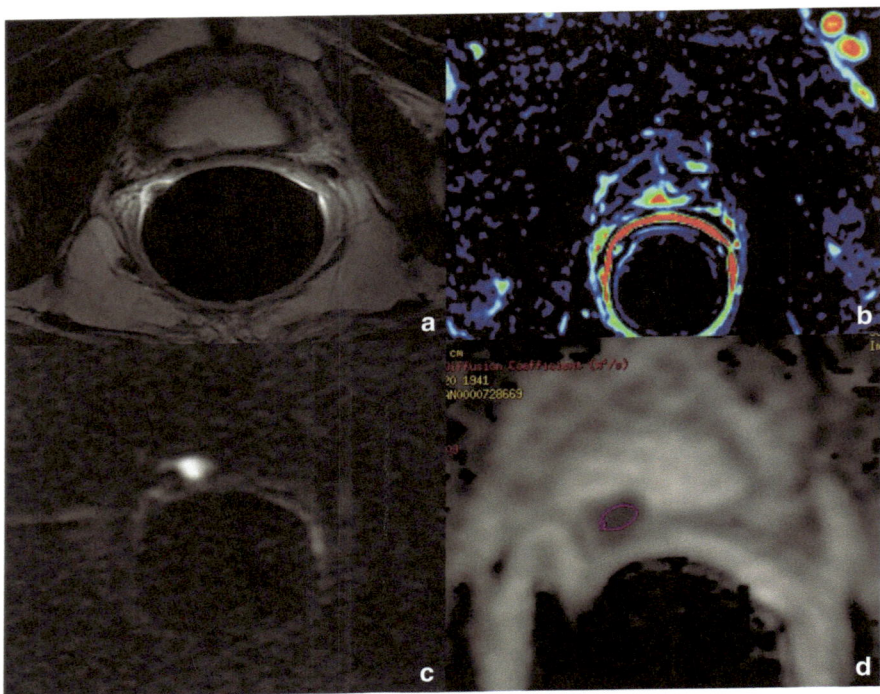

Fig. 8.3 Multiparametric-MR images of a 74-year-old man with prostate-specific antigen progression (PSA serum level 0.43 ng/ml) after radical retropubic prostatectomy, with suspected local recurrence. (**a**) Axial T2-weighted fast spin-echo image shows a solid nodular tissue of about 7 mm in size on the right posterior perianastomotic location in front of the rectal wall at about 12 mm from the ureteral meatus which is slightly hyperintense compared to pelvic muscles. (**b**) Axial Gradient-echo T1-weighted colour map image showing a remarkable enhancement of the pathological tissue. (**c**) Axial DWI image at b value $= 1,000$ s/mm showing marked restricted diffusion phenomena of water molecules. (**d**) Axial ADC map reconstructed from images obtained at b values of 0, 500 and 1,000 shows a *dark area* corresponding to the abnormal hyperintense tissue seen on T2-weighted images and hypervascular nodule seen on colour map. All these findings are consistent with locoregional relapse

recurrence, 1.1 ± 1.17 mm^2/s for low-grade aggressiveness relapse and the patients with a histological finding of residual glandular tissue had ADC values higher than 1.3 mm^2/s (mean ADC values 1.4; range 1.3–1.7).

The perianastomotic fibrosis appears hypointense on T2-weighted images, with absent enhancement on DCE-MRI. After DCE-MRI, all benign nodules show signal enhancement of less than 50 % in the early phase, whereas all recurrences showed fast signal enhancement in the early phase followed by a plateau or washout. Recurrences appear as masses with intermediate to high signal intensity on T2-weighted images compared to pelvic muscles, enhancing after intravenous injection of contrast medium.

In a single-centre retrospective study, Sella et al. [56] analysed 48 patients with biochemical progression after RP with a mean lesion size (maximum diameter) of

1.4 cm (range 0.8–4.5) and a mean PSA serum level of 2.18 ng/ml (range 0–10 ng/ml); the sensitivity and specificity of MRI were respectively 95 % and 100 %, but these results were achieved with a limited sample of patients and furthermore they rested on a too large size of local recurrence and a too high PSA values.

Following studies confirmed the importance of MRI in the depiction of local prostate cancer recurrence in patients with biochemical progression after RP.

Cirillo et al. [60] in a patient population of 72 units (range of local recurrence diameter: 0.8–3.5 cm, average 1.7 cm; mean PSA level 1.23 ± 1.3 ng/ml, range 0.2–8.8 ng/ml) compared T2-weighted to DCE images achieving a sensitivity, specificity and accuracy of 61.4 %, 82.1 % and 69.4 % for T2-weighted imaging and 84.1 %, 89.3 % and 86.1 % for DCE images.

Casciani et al. [57] in a single-centre retrospective study described the use of MRI with DCE in 46 patients who previously underwent RP (mean diameter of the lesion 1.5 cm with a range of 0.4–4.0 cm; mean PSA level 1.9 ng/ml, range 0.1–6.0 ng/ml) achieving a sensitivity, specificity and accuracy of 88 %, 100 % and 94 %.

Although these studies were based on a considerable number of patients and mean PSA level was not very high, they were partially limited by the average size of local recurrence always >1.5 cm in diameter.

Sciarra et al. [58], in a patient population of 70 units (mean PSA level in group A 1.26 ng/ml, in group B 0.8 ng/ml; mean lesion size 13.3 mm in group A and 6 mm in group B), compared 1H-MRSI and DCE-MRI showing a sensitivity of 71–84 % and a specificity of 83–88 % for 1H-MRSI alone, a sensitivity of 71–79 % and a specificity of 94–100 % for DCE-MRI alone; and for the two combined techniques a sensitivity of 86–87 % and specificity of 94–100 %.

A recent study [61] demonstrated, in a patient population of 84 units (mean PSA level 1.1 ng/ml in group A, 1.9 ng/ml in group B; mean lesion size 6 mm in group A, 13.3 mm in group B), that combined technique of 1H-MRSI and DCE-MRI at 3 T magnet is a valid tool to detect local prostate cancer recurrence and it is more accurate than Ch-PET/CT in the identification of small lesions in patients with low biochemical alterations after RP (PSA level: 0.2–2 ng/ml).

The last two studies were based on a solid number of patients and depicted tumour recurrences <1.5 cm in size, but they did not compare DCE-MRI with DWI.

Nowadays, there is an increasingly growing interest in DWI, due to its non-invasiveness, because it is an emergent technique that can be performed without the administration of exogenous contrast medium, being therefore the most practical and simple to use [62]. It is a powerful tool in detecting PC [63] and localising prostate cancer recurrence in patients with biochemical failure after definitive radiation therapy [64]. In a recent study, Gennarini et al. reported five patients with biochemical recurrence after RP and pelvic lymph node dissection in whom local recurrence could only be detected with DWI [65]. Recent studies demonstrate the usefulness of DWI technique in detecting local tumour recurrence after external beam radiation therapy [64] and after RP [65], even though these early experiences were based on a small number of cases.

Panebianco et al. [59], in a single-centre prospective study, analysed a large number of patients (262 consecutive male patients) in order to validate the role of 3-T DWI in mp-MRI in the detection of local prostate cancer recurrence in patients with biochemical progression of PSA serum level after RP. All in all, the accuracy of DWI was slightly lower than DCE (92 % versus 93 % in group A and 89 % versus 91 % in group B). The authors supposed that the overall accuracy of DCE imaging is superior to that of DWI because DW images are more affected by intrinsic distortion artefacts and background noise than DCE images are, though there are some cases in which DCE is doubtful and DWI is of primary importance for local recurrence depiction. For example, sometimes is very difficult to discriminate between prominent periprostatic venous plexus and enhancing recurrent tumour on the basis of DCE alone [66]; therefore, when there is this potential pitfall DWI is needful to exclude the presence of pathological tissue in post-prostatectomy bed. This experience highlights the diagnostic power of DW imaging almost comparable to DCE-MRI, this being up to now assumed as the most reliable MRI technique in detecting local prostate cancer recurrence, thus justifying an MRI imaging protocol of post-prostatectomy fossa consisting only of morphological T2-weigted images and DW imaging in patients with renal failure. Moreover, these results could pave the way to the possibility of using DWI as an alternative to DCE-MRI for follow-up after RP, with a high sensitivity, specificity and accuracy in detecting local recurrence. Besides, the possibility of using DWI as an alternative to DCE is supported thanks to its short acquisition time and repeatability, which are superior to that of DCE, and also because DWI is free from complications and danger given the absence of intravenous administration of contrast-medium.

Conclusions

Choline PET/CT is the most promising whole body imaging modality in detecting distant metastases of PC, because of its capability in detecting with high sensitivity small lymph node localisations or bone metastases, with a positive effect on general clinical management of PC patients and their prognosis, because of the intrinsic property of the tracer and the possibility to assess in a single session both metabolic and anatomic information about the disease.

This role can be enhanced by the adequate selection of the patients by means of PSA, PSA kinetics (such as PSAdt and PSAve), especially in those patients treated with surgical curative intent. Furthermore, the selection of the patients undergone to choline PET/CT must be take into account the possibility concurrent hormonal therapy, that could negatively affects the sensitivity of the exam. To date, the possible role of this diagnostic tool in detecting local relapse still remains unclear. The detection rate of PET/CT for local recurrence seems to be poor, probably because of PET spatial resolution (5–6 mm) which does not allow the depiction of small lesions.

Recently, mp-MRI more than other imaging procedures has been proposed as a useful tool in the diagnosing of local recurrence of prostate cancer after RP, but up to now it does not have a large availability in hospitals, it is a procedure that requires time and it does not have good detection rates for nodal and distant metastasis. At present, mp-MRI after RP is indicated to diagnose small local recurrence in a range of PSA serum level between 0.2 and 1 ng/ml when choline PET/CT is not suitable. Mp-MRI, thanks to functional imaging, allows also to distinguish between residual glandular tissue and or/fibrosis and nodule recurrence and it may also be able to determine the aggressiveness of nodule recurrence.

Future studies are needed to assess the performance of choline PET/CT in diagnosis of local relapse of PC; in particular, the recent development of hybrid PET/MRI scanners could improve the diagnosis of local relapse of PC in prostatic fossa.

References

1. Parker SL, Tong T, Bolden S, Wingo PA (1997) Cancer statistics, 1997. Cancer J Clin 47(1): 5–27
2. Bill-Axelson A, Holmberg L, Filén F et al (2008) Radical prostatectomy versus watchful waiting in localized prostate cancer: the Scandinavian prostate cancer group-4 randomized trial. J Natl Cancer Inst 100(16):1144–1154
3. Han M, Partin AW, Zahurak M, Piantadosi S, Epstein JI, Walsh PC (2003) Biochemical (prostate specific antigen) recurrence probability following radical prostatectomy for clinically localized prostate cancer. J Urol 169(2):517–523
4. Grossfeld GD, Stier DM, Flanders SC et al (1998) Use of second treatment following definitive local therapy for prostate cancer: data from the caPSURE database. J Urol 160:1398–1404
5. Freedland SJ, Humphreys EB, Mangold LA, Eisenberger M, Partin AW (2006) Time to prostate specific antigen recurrence after radical prostatectomy and risk of prostate cancer specific mortality. J Urol 176:1404–1408
6. Amling CL, Bergstralh EJ, Blute ML, Slezak JM, Zincke H (2001) Defining prostate specific antigen progression after radical prostatectomy: what is the most appropriate cut point? J Urol 165:1146–1151
7. Svatek R, Karakiewicz PI, Shulman M, Karam J, Perrotte P, Benaim E (2006) Pre-treatment nomogram for disease-specific survival of patients with chemotherapy-naive androgen independent prostate cancer. Eur Urol 49(4):666–674
8. EAU (2012) Guidelines on prostate cancer. European Association of Urology, Arnhem
9. Roberts SG, Blute ML, Bergstralh EJ, Slezak JM, Zincke H (2001) PSA doubling time as a predictor of clinical progression after biochemical failure following radical prostatectomy for prostate cancer. Mayo Clin Proc 76(6):576–581
10. Marks RA, Koch MO, Lopez-Beltran A, Montironi R, Juliar BE, Cheng L (2007) The relationship between the extent of surgical margin positivity and prostate specific antigen recurrence in radical prostatectomy specimens. Hum Pathol 38(8):1207–1211
11. Stephenson AJ, Scardino PT, Kattan MW et al (2007) Predicting the outcome of salvage radiation therapy for recurrent prostate cancer after radical prostatectomy. J Clin Oncol 25(15): 2035–2041
12. Loblaw D, Mendelson DS, Talcott JA et al (2004) American society of clinical oncology recommendations for the initial hormonal management of androgen sensitive metastatic, recurrent, or progressive prostate cancer. J Clin Oncol 22:2927–2941
13. Leventis AK, Shariat SF, Slawin KM (2001) Local recurrence after radical prostatectomy. Correlation of US features with prostatic fossa biopsy findings. Radiology 219:432–439
14. Scattoni V, Montorsi F, Picchio M, Roscigno M, Salonia A, Rigatti P et al (2004) Diagnosis of local recurrence after radical prostatectomy. BJU Int 93(5):680–688

15. Goldenberg SL, Carter M, Dashefsky S, Cooperberg PL (1992) Sonographic characteristics of the urethrovesical anastomosis in the early post-radical prostatectomy patient. J Urol 147:1307–1309
16. Picchio M, Crivellaro C, Giovacchini G, Gianolli L, Messa C (2009) PET-CT for treatment planning in prostate cancer. Q J Nucl Med Mol Imaging 53(2):245–268
17. Schillaci O, Calabria F, Tavolozza M, Cicciò C, Carlani M, Caracciolo CR et al (2010) 18F-choline PET/CT physiological distribution and pitfalls in image interpretation: experience in 80 patients with prostate cancer. Nucl Med Commun 31(1):39–45
18. Hara T, Kosaka N, Shinoura N, Kondo T (1997) PET imaging of brain tumor with [methyl-11C]choline. J Nucl Med 38:842–847
19. Khan N, Oriuchi N, Zhang H et al (2003) A comparative study of 11C-choline PET and [18F] fluorodeoxyglucose PET in the evaluation of lung cancer. Nucl Med Commun 24:359–366
20. Picchio M, Treiber U, Beer AJ et al (2006) Value of 11C-choline PET and contrast-enhanced CT for staging of bladder cancer: correlation with histopathologic findings. J Nucl Med 47:938–944
21. García JR, Soler M, Blanch MA, Ramírez I, Riera E, Lozano P et al (2009) PET/CT with (11) C-choline and (18)F-FDG in patients with elevated PSA after radical treatment of a prostate cancer. Rev Esp Med Nucl 28(3):95–100
22. Picchio M, Messa C, Landoni C et al (2003) Value of [11C]choline-positron emission tomography for re-staging prostate cancer: a comparison with [18F]fluorodeoxyglucose-positron emission tomography. J Urol 169:1337–1340
23. Scher B, Seitz M, Albinger W et al (2007) Value of 11C choline PET and PET/CT in patients with suspected prostate cancer. Eur J Nucl Med Mol Imaging 34:45–53
24. Giovacchini G, Picchio M, Coradeschi E et al (2008) [(11)C]choline uptake with PET/CT for the initial diagnosis of prostate cancer: relation to PSA levels, tumour stage and anti-androgenic therapy. Eur J Nucl Med Mol Imaging 35:1065–1073
25. Rinnab L, Blumstein NM, Mottaghy FM et al (2007) 11C choline positron-emission tomography/computed tomography and transrectal ultrasonography for staging localized prostate cancer. BJU Int 99:1421–1426
26. Schiavina R, Scattoni V, Castellucci P et al (2008) (11)C-choline positron emission tomography/computerized tomography for preoperative lymph-node staging in intermediate-risk and high-risk prostate cancer: comparison with clinical staging nomograms. Eur Urol 54:392–401
27. Calabria F, Chiaravalloti A, Tavolozza M, Ragano-Caracciolo C, Schillaci O (2013) Evaluation of extraprostatic disease in the staging of prostate cancer by F-18 choline PET/CT: can PSA and PSA density help in patient selection? Nucl Med Commun 2013 34(8):733–740
28. Heidenreich A, Aus G, Bolla M et al (2008) EAU guidelines on prostate cancer. Eur Urol 53:68–80
29. Fazio F, Picchio M, Messa C (2004) Is 11C-choline the most appropriate tracer for prostate cancer? Eur J Nucl Med Mol Imaging 31:753–756
30. Heinisch M, Dirisamer A, Loidl W et al (2006) Positron emission tomography/computed tomography with F-18-fluorocholine for restaging of prostate cancer patients: meaningful at PSA < 5 ng/ml? Mol Imaging Biol 8(1):43–48
31. Rinnab L, Mottaghy FM, Blumstein NM et al (2007) Evaluation of [11C]-choline positron-emission/computed tomography in patients with increasing prostate-specific antigen levels after primary treatment for prostate cancer. BJU Int 10(4):786–793
32. Rinnab L, Simon J, Hautmann RE et al (2009) (11)C-choline PET/CT in prostate cancer patients with biochemical recurrence after radical prostatectomy. World J Urol 27(5):619–625
33. Castellucci P, Fuccio C, Nanni C et al (2009) Influence of trigger PSA and PSA kinetics on 11C-choline PET/CT detection rate in patients with biochemical relapse after radical prostatectomy. J Nucl Med 50(9):1394–1400
34. Castellucci P, Fuccio C, Rubello D et al (2011) Is there a role for 11C-choline PET/CT in the early detection of metastatic disease in surgically treated prostate cancer patients with a mild PSA increase < 1.5 ng/ml? Eur J Nucl Med Mol Imaging 38(1):55–63

35. Giovacchini G, Picchio M, Scattoni V et al (2010) PSA doubling time for prediction of [(11)C] choline PET/CT findings in prostate cancer patients with biochemical failure after radical prostatectomy. Eur J Nucl Med Mol Imaging 37(6):1106–1116

36. Giovacchini G, Picchio M, Briganti A et al (2010) [11C]-choline positron emission tomography/computerized tomography to restage prostate cancer cases with biochemical failure after radical prostatectomy and no disease evidence on conventional imaging. J Urol 184(3): 938–943

37. Giovacchini G, Picchio M, Coradeschi E et al (2010) Predictive factors of (11)C-choline PET/CT in patients with biochemical failure after radical prostatectomy. Eur J Nucl Med Mol Imaging 37(2):301–309

38. Reske SN, Blumstein NM, Glatting G (2008) [11C]-choline PET/CT imaging in occult local relapse of prostate cancer after radical prostatectomy. Eur J Nucl Med Mol Imaging 35(1): 9–17

39. Cimitan M, Bortolus R, Morassut S, Canzonieri V, Garbeglio A, Baresic T et al (2006) [18F] fluorocholine PET/CT imaging for the detection of recurrent prostate cancer at PSA relapse: experience in 100 consecutive patients. Eur J Nucl Med Mol Imaging 33(12):1387–1398

40. Krause BJ, Souvatzoglou M, Tuncel M et al (2008) The detection rate of (11)C-Choline-PET/CT depends on the serum PSA-value in patients with biochemical recurrence of prostate cancer. Eur J Nucl Med Mol Imaging 35:18–23

41. Giovacchini G, Picchio M, Parra RG, Briganti A, Gianolli L, Montorsi F et al (2012) Prostate-specific antigen velocity versus prostate-specific antigen doubling time for prediction of 11C choline PET/CT in prostate cancer patients with biochemical failure after radical prostatectomy. Clin Nucl Med 37(4):325–331

42. Winter A, Uphoff J, Henke RP, Wawroschek F (2010) First results of [11C]-choline PET/CT-guided secondary lymph node surgery in patients with PSA failure and single lymph node recurrence after radical retropubic prostatectomy. Urol Int 84(4):418–423

43. Wo JY, Chen MH, Nguyen PL, Renshaw AA, Loffredo MJ, Kantoff PW et al (2009) Evaluating the combined effect of comorbidity and prostate-specific antigen kinetics on the risk of death in men after prostate-specific antigen recurrence. J Clin Oncol 27(35):6000–6005

44. Benchikh E, Fegoun A, Villers A, Moreau JL, Richaud P, Rebillard X et al (2008) PSA and follow-up after treatment of prostate cancer. Prog Urol 18(3):137–144

45. Partin AW, Pearson JD, Landis PK, Carter HB, Pound CR, Clemens JQ et al (1994) Evaluation of serum prostate-specific antigen velocity after radical prostatectomy to distinguish local recurrence from distant metastases. Urology 43(5):649–659

46. Schillaci O, Calabria F, Tavolozza M, Caracciolo CR, Finazzi Agrò E, Miano R et al (2012) Influence of PSA, PSA velocity and PSA doubling time on contrast-enhanced 18F-choline PET/CT detection rate in patients with rising PSA after radical prostatectomy. Eur J Nucl Med Mol Imaging 39(4):589–596

47. Picchio M, Briganti A, Fanti S et al (2011) The role of choline positron emission tomography/computed tomography in the management of patients with prostate-specific antigen progression after radical treatment of prostate cancer. Eur Urol 59(1):51–60

48. Knopp MV, Giesel FL, Marcos H, von Tengg-Kobligk H, Choyke P (2001) Dynamic contrast-enhanced magnetic resonance imaging in oncology. Top Magn Reson Imaging 12(4):301–308

49. Seitz M, Shukla-Dave A, Bjartell A et al (2009) Functional magnetic resonance imaging in prostate cancer. Eur Urol 55(4):801–814

50. Fuchsjäger M, Akin O, Shukla-Dave A, Pucar D, Hricak H (2009) The role of MRI and MRSI in diagnosis, treatment selection, and post-treatment follow-up for prostate cancer. Clin Adv Hematol Oncol 7(3):193–202

51. Scattoni V, Montorsi F, Picchio M, Roscigno M, Salonia A, Rigatti P et al (2004) Diagnosis of local recurrence after radical prostatectomy. BJU Int 93(5):680–688

52. Alfarone A, Panebianco V, Schillaci O, Salciccia S, Cattarino S, Mariotti G et al (2012) Comparative analysis of multiparametric magnetic resonance and PET-CT in the management

of local recurrence after radical prostatectomy for prostate cancer. Crit Rev Oncol Hematol 84 (1):109–121

53. Kluwer W (2007) Perez and Brady's principles and practice of radiation oncology, 5th edn. Lippincott Williams & Wilkins, Philadelphia

54. Somford DM, Fütterer JJ, Hambrock T, Barentsz JO (2008) Diffusion and perfusion MR imaging of the prostate. Magn Reson Imaging Clin N Am 16(4):685–695

55. Fuccio C, Rubello D, Castellucci P, Marzola MC, Fanti S (2011) Choline PET/CT for prostate cancer: main clinical applications. Eur J Radiol 80(2):50–56

56. Sella T, Schwartz LH, Swindle PW et al (2004) Suspected local recurrence after radical prostatectomy: endorectal coil MR imaging. Radiology 231(2):379–385

57. Casciani E, Polettini E, Carmenini E et al (2008) Endorectal and dynamic contrast-enhanced MRI for detection of local recurrence after radical prostatectomy. AJR Am J Roentgenol 190 (5):1187–1192

58. Sciarra A, Panebianco V, Salciccia S et al (2008) Role of dynamic contrast-enhanced magnetic resonance (MR) imaging and proton MR spectroscopic imaging in the detection of local recurrence after radical prostatectomy for prostate cancer. Eur Urol 54(3):589–600

59. Panebianco V, Barchetti F, Sciarra A, Musio D, Forte V, Gentile V et al (2013) Prostate cancer recurrence after radical prostatectomy: the role of 3-T diffusion imaging in multi-parametric magnetic resonance imaging. Eur Radiol 23(6):1745–1752

60. Cirillo S, Petracchini M, Scotti L et al (2009) Endorectal magnetic resonance imaging at 1.5 Tesla to assess local recurrence following radical prostatectomy using T2-weighted and contrast-enhanced imaging. Eur Radiol 19(3):761–769

61. Panebianco V, Sciarra A, Lisi D et al (2012) Prostate cancer: 1HMRS-DCEMR at 3T versus [(18)F]choline PET/CT in the detection of local prostate cancer recurrence in men with biochemical progression after radical retropubic prostatectomy (RRP). Eur J Radiol 81 (4):700–708

62. Somford DM, Fütterer JJ, Hambrock T, Barentsz JO (2008) Diffusion and perfusion MR imaging of the prostate. Magn Reson Imaging Clin N Am 16(4):685–695

63. Kilinç R, Doluoglu OG, Sakman B, Ciliz DS, Yüksel E, Adasan O et al (2012) The correlation between diffusion-weighted imaging an histopathological evaluation of 356 prostate biopsy sites in patients with prostatic diseases. Urology. doi:10.5402/2012/252846

64. Morgan VA, Riches SF, Giles S, Dearnaley D, de Souza NM (2012) Diffusion-weighted MRI for locally recurrent prostate cancer after external beam radiotherapy. AJR Am J Roentgenol 198(3):596–602

65. Giannarini G, Nguyen DP, Thalmann GN, Thoeny HC (2012) Diffusion-weighted magnetic resonance imaging detects local recurrence after radical prostatectomy: initial experience. Eur Urol 61(3):616–620

66. Vargas HA, Wassberg C, Akin O, Hricak H (2012) MR imaging of treated prostate cancer. Radiology 262(1):26–42

Intermittent Androgen Deprivation in the New Era: The Role of Urologist and Oncologist in a Multidisciplinary Team (MDT)

Andrea Alfarone and Flavia Longo

9.1 Introduction and Preliminary Considerations

Androgen deprivation therapy (ADT) for prostate cancer was first described in 1941 by Huggins and Hodges [1, 2]. They demonstrated the effect of surgical castration and oestrogen administration on the progression of metastatic *prostate cancer* (PC). Since then, androgen-suppressing strategies have become the mainstay of management of advanced PC. More recently, there has been a move towards the increasing use of hormonal treatment in younger men with earlier disease (i.e. non-metastatic) or recurrent disease after definitive treatment, either as primary single-agent therapy or as a part of a multimodality approach [3].

Prostate cells are physiologically dependent on androgens to stimulate growth, function, and proliferation. Testosterone, although not tumorigenic, is essential for the growth and perpetuation of tumour cells [4]. The testes are the source of most androgens, with adrenal biosynthesis providing only 5–10 % of androgens (i.e. androstenedione, dehydroepiandrosterone, and dehydroepiandrosterone sulphate).

Testosterone secretion is regulated by the hypothalamic–pituitary–gonadal axis. Within the prostate cell, testosterone is converted to 5-α-dihydrotestosterone (DHT) by the enzyme 5-α-reductase; DHT is an androgenic stimulant about 10 times more powerful than testosterone. Meanwhile, circulating testosterone is peripherally aromatized and converted to oestrogens, which together with circulating androgens, exert a negative feedback control on hypothalamic luteinizing hormone (LH) secretion.

If prostate cells are deprived of androgenic stimulation, they undergo apoptosis. Any treatment that results ultimately in suppression of androgen activity is referred to as ADT. Androgen deprivation can be achieved by either suppressing the secretion of testicular androgens by surgical or medical castration or inhibiting

A. Alfarone (✉) • F. Longo
Department of Urology, University Sapienza Rome, Viale del Policlinico 155, Rome 00144, Italy
e-mail: alfarone2@hotmail.com

V. Gentile et al. (eds.), *Multidisciplinary Management of Prostate Cancer*, 105
DOI 10.1007/978-3-319-04385-2_9, © Springer International Publishing Switzerland 2014

the action of circulating androgens at the level of their receptor in prostate cells using competing compounds known as antiandrogens. In addition, these two methods of androgen deprivation can be combined to achieve what is commonly known as *complete (or maximal or total) androgen blockade* (CAB).

Surgical castration is still considered the "gold standard" for ADT, against which all other treatments are rated. Removal of the testicular source of androgens leads to a considerable decline in testosterone levels and induces a hypogonadal status, although a very low level of testosterone (known as the "castration level") persists.

The standard castrate level is <50 ng/dl. It was defined more than 40 years ago, when testosterone level testing was limited. However, current testing methods using chemiluminescence have found that the mean value of testosterone after surgical castration is 15 ng/dl [5].

Bilateral orchiectomy, which is either total or sub-capsular (i.e. with preservation of tunica albuginea and epididymis), is a simple and virtually complication-free surgical procedure. It is easily performed under local anaesthesia [6] and is the quickest way to achieve a castration level, usually within less than 12 h.

The main drawback of orchiectomy is that it may have a negative psychological effect: some men consider it to be an unacceptable assault on their manhood. In addition, it is irreversible and does not allow for *intermittent treatment*. The use of oestrogens, LHRH agonists, and LHRH antagonists are all methods to achieve androgen deprivation with the aim to reach surgical castration level of testosterone [7–9]. In the last 20 years, the LHRH agonists have largely replaced surgical castration.

The appeal of the agonists is their reversibility. Data on the adverse systemic effects of ADT have increasingly emerged since the early 2000s. Androgen deprivation therapy is associated with *multiple side effects*, including hot flushes, decreased energy, loss of libido, erectile dysfunction, cognitive dysfunction, fatigue, depression, osteoporosis, changes in body composition, gynaecomastia, anaemia, and a form of metabolic syndrome characterized by abdominal obesity and insulin resistance that increases the risk of cardiovascular events [10, 11]. The increased recognition of those side effects enhanced the appeal of reducing patient exposure to ADT.

This was one of the reasons why the concept of *intermittent androgen deprivation* (IAD) was introduced, based on alternating periods of hormonal therapy and cessation of treatment, allowing for hormonal recovery and, thus, reducing unwanted side effects. The second reason for IAD therapy is the possibility of delaying also the condition of hormone refractory cancer as a final stage of the natural history of the disease. This phenomenon was well demonstrated in a preclinical study published by Bruchovsky et al. where they found a 500-fold increase of androgen-independent cells in proportion to 20 times androgen-dependent cells after castration in animal models (Shionogi mice) [12]. Akakura et al. also showed that the period of progression to a castration resistant prostate cancer (CRPC) was 3 times higher for the IAD than for the continuous [13].

Apparently, androgen suppression in some moment and due to unknown causes would lead the prostate stem cell to a state of hormone insensitivity; therefore, disrupting the androgen suppression "temporarily" would help keep the tumour sensitive [14].

Klotz et al. were the ones who developed and published the first clinical study in 1986 using the IAD as a treatment [15]. It consisted in the discontinuation of diethylstilbestrol in patients with metastatic PC after manifesting an objective clinical response to the treatment. Once the patients began again with symptoms resulting from PC, the treatment was restarted again, reporting a rapid clinical response again. The principle of IAD is that when a predetermined *PSA nadir* is reached, hormone treatment can be stopped. Treatment is restarted once the PSA rises to a predetermined level or when there is evidence of clinical progression. Approximately 95 % of patients diagnosed with prostate cancer can be expected to show a PSA response adequate to allow cessation of hormone therapy. This proportion decreases with each successive cycle of hormone therapy. Those patients who fail to achieve an adequate nadir level have the poorest prognosis and require prolonged hormone therapy and consideration for second-line hormone therapy and/or chemotherapy.

PSA is the marker used to monitor response in IAD protocols. PSA production is androgen dependent. Frequently studies using PSA as an outcome do not include data on testosterone levels. Interpretation of PSA levels in the absence of contemporaneous serum testosterone is of limited value. PSA is currently the best marker as its measurement is easy and universally available. A consistent rise in PSA despite castrate levels of androgens is considered to indicate the onset of androgen independent growth.

IAD is a *cyclic therapy* consisting of on-treatment periods followed by off-treatment periods. A complete IAD cycle comprises both the on- and off-treatment periods and is thus the period between initiating hormonal therapy and reinstituting treatment after an off-treatment period [16].

Treatment can consist of CAD or LHRH agonist monotherapy and should ideally be continued until castration-induced apoptosis is maximal and tumour regression is induced, but it should be stopped before the androgen-independent phenotype is developed [17, 18].

Caution is warranted in patients with high pre-treatment PSA levels or low PSA doubling times, patients with a high clinical stage or high-grade disease, or patients with a high metastatic burden [18–20]. Numerous studies in recent years have outlined the main criteria that must be followed during IAD treatment.

9.2 Phase II Studies

Many prospective trials on IAD were reported. Most were phase II or retrospective, and also single-institution series with relatively small numbers of patients. All phase II trials have extremely heterogeneous design with respect to patients, PSA cut-off, cycle lengths, and treatment regimen, making comparisons difficult. Regimens generally used an LHRH agonist with or without an antiandrogen.

In the off-treatment interval, quality of life was consistently improved, although most of the studies failed to use validated quality of life instruments. Most trials included patients with a mix of disease stages, from biochemical recurrence, to local recurrence, to metastatic disease.

An overview of the phase II IAD studies estimated the 5-year *overall survival* to be 86 % in men with biochemical recurrence, 68 % in men with metastatic disease, and 90 % in men with localized disease [21]. Development of early castration resistant disease was a relatively rare event [22]. The studies identified a number of prognostic factors for time to androgen-independent progression. Those factors included duration of the off-treatment interval, baseline PSA, and PSA nadir. In a large prospective Canadian trial, the time-off treatment averaged 53 % of the total cycle time, but in absolute terms, it declined with each succeeding cycle, ranging from 63.7 weeks in cycle 1 to 25.6 weeks in cycle 5 [23–27]. Of course, none of the trials was able to address the key question of the impact of IAD on survival.

The level of *testosterone* recovery was discussed in about 60 % of studies; where reported, the proportion of men in whom serum testosterone normalized was generally high following the first cycle (in the region of 70–90 %) but tended to decrease during subsequent cycles. Factors influencing time to delay in testosterone normalization may include advanced age, low baseline testosterone levels, and duration of ADT [26, 27]. Bruchovsky et al. [23] also identified a close relationship between the recoveries of serum testosterone and PSA: men who quickly recovered serum testosterone experienced a more rapid rise in serum PSA levels and a shorter time-off therapy.

Shaw et al. [21] in their very interesting meta-analysis described that patients on IAD spent a mean of 39 % of time-off treatment. Multivariate models showed as predicting factors, the initial PSA level and PSA nadir, the type of treatment and the PSA threshold for restarting treatment. CAD or LHRH analogue should be the standard for patients treated with IAD.

9.3   Phase III Studies

Several phase III trials have been recently reported that address several unanswered questions on IAD (Table 9.1). Some of these have reported survival data [28–30] and showed no difference in overall and prostate Cancer-specific survival between groups. There are important differences among the randomized phase III studies on IAD. The cohort sizes are modest in the study by de Leval et al. [31] and in the TULP [32] and TAP22 [28] trials. In contrast, the SEUG 9401 [33], SWOG 9346 [30], NCT3653 [29], and FinnProstate VII [34] studies were performed with significant numbers of patients with extended follow-up. However, some of these last studies (SEUG 9401 and FinnProstate VII) included mixed populations, and this is a relevant disadvantage when compared with trials including only pure cohorts (SWOG 9346 and NCT3653).

Table 9.1 Population characteristics in phase III trials

	De Leval [31]	TAP 22 [28]	TULP [32]	FINN Prostate [34]	SEUG 9401 [33]	NCT 3653 [29]	SWOG 9346 [30]	SEUG 9901 [37]
Number of cases	68	173	193	554	766	1,386	1,535	1,045
Tumour stage	Locally advanced/ Metastatic/ Biochemical recurrence	Metastatic	Metastatic	Locally advanced/ Metastatic	Locally advanced/ Metastatic	After radiotherapy	Metastatic	Locally advanced/ Metastatic
PSA at inclusion	Any value	>20 ng/ml	Any value	Any value	>4 and < 100 ng/ml	>3 ng/ml	>5 ng/ml	>4 and < 100 ng/ml
Induction period (months)	6	6	6	6	3	8	7	3
PSA level to stop On-treatment	<4 ng/ml	<4 ng/ml	<4 ng/ml	<10 ng/ml	<4 ng/ml	<4 ng/ml	<4 ng/ml	<4 ng/ml
PSA level to start On-treatment	>10 ng/ml	>10 ng/ml	>10 ng/ml not metastatic to >20 metastatic	>20 ng/ml	>10 for symptomatic >20 ng for asymptomatic	>10 ng/ml	>20 ng/ml	>20 ng/ml
Time-off therapy	3.3–8.3 months	1.0–48.9 months	0.7–4.9 months	10.9–33.5 weeks	50 % at least 52 weeks; 29 % for 36 months	20–59.6 months	>40 % of time	50 % after 2.5 years and 28 % after 5 years
Follow-up (months)	31	44	31	65	50	84	108	66

Most of the phase III trials tended to focus on advanced or metastatic disease rather than biochemical failure, except for the NCT3653 trial [29] and others not yet published [35].

Although there was apparent consensus in most trials on the PSA level designated for *ADT discontinuation* (<4 ng/ml), the criteria for resuming treatment were less uniform (>10 ng/ml or >20 ng/ml, depending on the stage and the presence of symptoms) [22].

Time-off therapy is variable in the different studies (from 0.7–4.9 months in the TULP study to 20–59.6 months in the NCT3653 study), and the risk is that in some studies, IAD patients are often on therapy rather than off. In particular, the duration of off-treatment periods decreased progressively during the following cycles of IAD. The conclusions of these trials support the hypothesis that IAD, mainly in metastatic cases, can produce oncologic results similar (not inferior, as defined by some trials) to those of continuous ADT.

Although many studies and publications evaluated the efficacy of IAD, the evaluation of the *safety and tolerability* of this regimen is often limited, and data are not complete in all respects. Early side effects as hot flushes and sexual dysfunction are the most common early side effects described during ADT and are able to affect patient quality of life (QoL) [36].

In the TAP22 trial [28], the incidence of adverse side effects was significantly higher in the continuous ADT group (93.6 %) than in the IAD group (84.4 %) ($p = 0.042$). In the TULP trial [32], a trend of more side effects like hot flushes was seen in the continuous ADT group compared with the IAD group.

In the NCT3653 trial [29], IAD was associated with significantly better scores (not specified; $p < 0.001$) for hot flushes and desire for sexual activity. Although only 35 % of patients in the IAD group had a return to pre-treatment testosterone levels within 2 years after completing the first period of treatment, 79 % had a level of at least 5 nmol/l.

In the study by de Leval et al. [31], hot flushes were reported as less frequent (not specified) and as mild to moderate during IAD treatment and were resolved or improved in the off-treatment periods. Regarding erectile dysfunction, lower incidence (not specified) was reported in the IAD group, with significant improvement during the off phases of treatment.

In the FinnProstate study [34], a non-significantly lower incidence ($p = 0.44$) of hot flushes was found for the IAD group. The only significant difference in early side effects emerged unexpectedly in the numbers of patients reporting erectile dysfunction and depression, which were more common in the IAD group (for IAD vs. continuous ADT, respectively, erectile dysfunction was reported by 15.7 % vs. 7.9 % and depression was reported by 2.2 % vs. 0 %; $p < 0.05$). In the IAD group, testosterone levels showed recovery at the end of each off-treatment phase but did not reach the same level as at the end of the previous off phases. At entry, 81.2 % of patients in the IAD arm had a *testosterone level* >10 nmol/l; however, only 47.4 % had a testosterone level >10 nmol/l at the end of the 10th off-treatment phase.

In the SEUG 9401 trial [33], patients on IAD experienced lower incidence of hot flushes and fewer problems related to *sexual function* and reported increased sexual activity ($p < 0.01$). In the first period after randomization, virtually all IAD patients were off therapy, and their levels of sexual activity were similar to pre-treatment levels (35 %). As the follow-up time increased, more IAD patients were on therapy and sexual activity decreased.

Long-term side effects of ADT include loss of bone mineral density, metabolic changes, and cardiovascular disease [36]. Publications related to phase III trials were not designed to examine the long-term consequences of ADT for these parameters. The SEUG 9401 trial [33] found an increased risk of dying from cardiovascular disease in the continuous ADT group (cardiovascular deaths: 41 [13.1 %] in the IAD group, 52 [16.7 %] in the continuous ADT group) but similar incidence of cardiac ischemia/infarction in both treatment arms (10 % for IAD, 11 % for continuous ADT).

In the FinnProstate study [34], no significant differences were found between the two treatment groups in terms of *cardiovascular side effects* (31.8 % for IAD vs. 33.9 % for continuous ADT; $p = 0.59$). Cardiovascular-related mortality was also similar (12.8 % for IAD vs. 15.4 % for continuous ADT; $p = 0.38$).

Only the Finn Prostate phase III trial [34] published a study specifically focused on the effect of IAD on QoL and adverse events. Based on available data, the frequency of early side effects such as hot flushes or sexual dysfunction significantly decreases in the IAD group when compared with the continuous-treatment group. The severity of early side effects was also improved in the IAD group.

Considering the QoL difference as a whole, the two treatment regimens seem to be very similar. Results are probably influenced by the duration of the off-treatment periods and by the rate of testosterone recovery.

A recent randomized phase III trial, the SEUG 9901 [37], demonstrated the non-inferiority of *antiandrogen monotherapy* in IAD compared with maximal androgen blockade. They enrolled 1,045 patients with locally advanced or metastatic prostate cancer, 918 responded to induction therapy and therefore were randomized. Overall survival (OS) was similar in the two groups, and non-inferiority of IAD was demonstrated with HR 0.90 (95 % CI 0.76–1.07). There was a trend for an interaction between treatment and PSA, favouring IAD over CAB in patients with PSA < 1 ng/ml. After randomization, 50 % of patients were off therapy for >2.5 years and 28 % were off therapy for >5 years. In IAD group were found better results on sexual function.

The two largest phase III trials to date are the NCT3653 study [29] and the SWOG 9346 [30]. Both were designed as non-inferiority studies. The results, which are somewhat contradictory, are intriguing. The NCT3653 trial enrolled 1,386 patients with a PSA level greater than 3 ng/ml more than 1 year after primary or salvage radiotherapy for localized PC. IAD was provided in 8-month cycles, with non-treatment periods determined according to the PSA level. The primary end point was *overall survival*. Secondary end points included *quality of life*, time to CRPC, and duration of non-treatment intervals. Median follow-up was 6.9 years. In the IAD group, full testosterone recovery occurred in 35 % of patients, and testosterone recovery to the trial-entry threshold occurred in 79 %. Patients on the intermittent arm were on treatment only 27 % of the time. Clear cut QOL benefits during the off-treatment interval were seen in the domains of erectile function, libido, hot flashes, physical function, fatigue, and urinary symptoms. There were 268 deaths in the intermittent-therapy group and 256 in the continuous-therapy group. Median overall survival was 8.8 years in the intermittent-therapy group versus 9.1 years in the continuous-therapy group (hazard ratio 1.02; 95 % CI 0.86–1.21). The 7-year cumulative rates of PC mortality were 18 % and 15 %, respectively ($p = 0.24$). This important study demonstrated that overall survival was equivalent in men with biochemical failure treated with intermittent therapy.

SWOG 9346 was designed to evaluate overall and disease-specific survival in IAD compared to continuous therapy, but in men with metastatic disease. A total of 1,535 patients with metastatic PC and a PSA > 5 ng/ml were submitted to 7 months of Goserelin and Bicalutamide. If the PSA was <4 ng/ml by month 6, they were then randomized between IAD and continuous therapy. Treatment was re-initiated when the PSA reached 20 ng/ml, and discontinued again after 7 months if the PSA was <4 ng/ml. Overall survival showed a non-significant trend to improvement in the continuous arm (HR 1.10, 95 % CI 0.99–1.23). However, considering HR values, the study was considered statistically inconclusive in terms to define a non-inferiority or an inferiority of IAD versus continuous CAD. Median survival was 5.8 vs. 5.1 years in IAD and continuous ADT, respectively. A sub-analysis stratifying by minimal disease (confined to axial skeleton and pelvis or lymph nodes) vs. extensive disease (ribs, long bones, skull, and/or viscera) was performed. This showed a benefit in the minimal disease group with continuous therapy, with a HR of 1.19, (95 % CI 0.98–1.43, $p = 0.034$) and none in the extensive disease group, with a HR of 1.02 (95 % CI 0.85–1.22). In the minimal disease group, median overall survival was 5.4 years in the IAD group vs. 6.9 years in the continuous group. The interpretation of this study is controversial. The stratification analysis was post hoc, and is therefore hypothesis generating, not proof, but also it is a challenge to make biological sense of the bracketing of the supposed inferiority of IAD in minimal metastatic disease, but not in non-metastatic or extensive metastatic disease.

9.4   Who Are Candidates for IAD

Some authors have suggested that poor candidates for IAD are those with initial bulky tumour, numerous positive lymph nodes or bone metastases, PSA doubling time (PSADT) <9 months and initial serum PSA >100 ng/ml, or severe pain [22, 38, 39]. The failure to achieve a low *nadir PSA* should preclude intermittent therapy. Similarly, patients with rapidly *rising PSA* (>5 ng/ml per month) or persistent pain from bone metastases are poor candidates for IAD [34, 40]. Other authors [41] have suggested that the best candidates for IAD are those patients with biochemical failure and rapidly rising PSA after radiotherapy or surgery. Gleave et al. [18] suggested that patients who failed to achieve a PSA nadir of <4 ng/ml after the induction period of 6 months should not be offered IAD. Pre-treatment variables such as tumour stage or grade can influence IAD results. In clinical practice, the characteristics of the *first cycle* of IAD could be used to predict response and select patients for further withdrawal of therapy; however, evidence is available only from phase II studies. The PSA nadir after initiating therapy and the rate of recovery of PSA during the first off-treatment interval are useful parameters. The criteria to define a clear response using these parameters are still pending, and we do not have any randomized trial focused on this point. Patients who are not good candidates for IAD generally declare themselves, either by having a poor PSA response to ADT (i.e. failure of PSA to drop to undetectable or very low levels) or a very rapid rise in PSA during the off-treatment interval. Even in high-risk patients without metastatic disease, an initial trial of discontinuing therapy in those whose PSA drops dramatically is appealing and carries little risk. Based on the SWOG study results in metastatic disease, caution is warranted in men with bone metastases. These men have a shorter life expectancy and shorter mean *off-treatment intervals*. Some metastatic patients, however, demonstrate a sustained and complete response to ADT. The nadir PSA on treatment is a predictor for the duration of response. A practical approach is to initiate ADT therapy, and reassess the patient based on their PSA and clinical response. Those patients with a complete biochemical response (PSA undetectable) should be considered for IAD. Should the off-treatment interval prove to be short due to rapid PSA recovery, these patients would be quickly restarted back on continuous therapy. Some patients, however, will have the benefit of a prolonged off-treatment interval despite the presence of bone metastasis and would benefit from this approach.

9.5 Trigger Points

Different durations of induction ADT are currently being compared. It takes 8–9 months to achieve a PSA nadir on average. More prolonged ADT results in permanent testosterone suppression. Thus, an 8–9-month period of ADT induction seems reasonable.

Most trials required a PSA drop to <4 ng/ml before discontinuing ADT. The usual PSA trigger for re-treatment was a PSA between 10 and 20 ng/ml. One meta-analysis of the phase II trials demonstrated improved survival when the PSA threshold for restarting treatment was <15 ng/ml [21].

Most phase III trials with published results used the combination of an LHRH agonist and short-term antiandrogen for flare blockade. The role of combined androgen blockade in intermittent therapy is unclear. Flare blockade is appropriate given the short duration of treatment. Some modelling of prostate cancer kinetics suggests that more aggressive hormonal blockade during the on treatment interval is of benefit, but this has yet to be demonstrated in clinical practice.

LHRH antagonists may result in more prompt testosterone recovery in the *off-treatment interval*, which would be advantageous in IAD.

PSA nadir after ADT is a strong predictor of progression [29, 42]. Patients whose PSA remained detectable on ADT had a 15 times greater likelihood of progressing to CRPC within 24 months, compared to those with an undetectable PSA [43]. A PSA nadir after the first cycle of <0.1 ng/ml is favourable, while failure to nadir below 0.4 ng/ml is associated with a two to threefold risk of CRPC and clinical progression [44]. The duration of the off-treatment cycle also predicts for *time to progression*. A shorter off-treatment cycle confers a relative risk for progression to CRPC and death of three to four [44, 45]. One of the advantages of intermittent therapy is that one can infer prognosis and allow identification of patients at higher risk of progression. This becomes relevant as new therapies for advanced PC emerge.

Testosterone recovery drives quality of life improvement during the off-treatment interval. This recovery rate is variable. Factors that influence testosterone recovery include the duration of the ADT induction period, the number of prior ADT cycles, age, baseline testosterone, and ethnicity [32]. In the Canadian phase II study, most patients recovered testosterone by 5 months in the first cycle [24]. Recovery of serum testosterone to a level of > or = 7.5 nmol/L was observed in 75 %, 50 %, 40 %, and 30 % of men in cycles 1 to 4, respectively. The off-treatment interval in the phase III trials ranged from 50–82 % [28, 32, 33, 46]. It was 73 % in the NCT3653 trial [29]. Most studies have shown that the duration of the off-treatment interval diminishes with successive cycles (in spite of the slower recovery of testosterone). This likely reflects the acquisition of a *castration-resistant phenotype*, with PSA recovery at lower levels of androgen. Thus, patients must be monitored closely for PSA and testosterone at least every 3 months while off treatment.

Conclusions

Data suggest that IAD can produce oncologic results similar (not inferior, as defined by some trials) to those of continuous ADT but with potentially better tolerability. We need more studies to create correct guidelines about IAD treatment. It is fundamental to find exact trigger points for all situations, in particular for patients with metastatic disease. Better stratification of results is needed in terms of prognostic parameters such as disease extension and Gleason score. Moreover, data are still insufficient to determine whether IAD is able to prevent long-term complications related to ADT. Comparative studies focused on QoL are warranted. It would also be interesting to analyze in depth differences between these two therapeutic approaches in terms of costs. In a recent review, Niraula et al. demonstrated that there is a median saving cost of about 48 % with IAD [47]. Therefore, we are waiting for more data to better select patient with PC to submit to IAD therapy. For all these reasons, the role of Urologist and Oncologist can be considered overlapping when we talk about IAD. In our opinion, a multidisciplinary approach is the best way not only to choose the exact therapeutic treatment but also to choose the best follow-up and to manage all complications of patients who may remain in therapy for many years.

References

1. Huggins C, Hodges CV (2002) Studies on prostatic cancer: I. The effect of castration, of estrogen and of androgen injection on serum phosphatases in metastatic carcinoma of the prostate, 1941. J Urol 168:9–12
2. Huggins C, Stevens RE Jr, Hodges CV (1941) Studies on prostate cancer. II. The effect of castration on advanced carcinoma of the prostate gland. Arch Surg 43:209–223
3. McLeod DG (2003) Hormonal therapy: historical perspective to future directions. Urology 61 (2 Suppl 1):3–7
4. Walsh PC (1975) Physiologic basis for hormonal therapy in carcinoma of the prostate. Urol Clin North Am 2(1):125–140
5. Efelein MG, Feng A, Scolieri MJ et al (2000) Reassessment of the definition of castrate levels of testosterone: implications for clinical decision making. Urology 56(6):1021–1024
6. Desmond AD, Arnold AJ, Hastie KJ (1988) Subcapsular orchiectomy under local anaesthesia. Technique, results and implications. Br J Urol 61(2):143–145
7. Limonta P, Montagnani MM, Moretti RM (2001) LHRH analogues as anticancer agents: pituitary and extrapituitary sites of action. Expert Opin Investig Drugs 10(4):709–720
8. Klotz L, Boccon-Gibod L, Shore ND et al (2008) The efficacy and safety of degarelix: a 12-month, comparative, randomized, open-label, parallel-group phase III study in patients with prostate cancer. BJU Int 102(11):1531–1538
9. Crawford ED, Tombal B, Miller K et al (2011) A phase III extension trial with a 1-arm crossover from leuprolide to degarelix: comparison of gonadotropin-releasing hormone agonist and antagonist effect on prostate cancer. J Urol 186(3):889–897
10. Higano CS (2003) Side effects of androgen deprivation therapy: monitoring and minimizing toxicity. Urology 61(suppl 1):32–38
11. Azoulay L, Yin H, Benayoun S et al (2011) Androgen-deprivation therapy and the risk of stroke in patients with prostate cancer. Eur Urol 60:1244–1250
12. Bruchovsky N, Rennie PS, Coldman AJ et al (1990) Effects of androgen withdrawal on the stem cell composition of the Shionogi carcinoma. Cancer Res 50:2275–2282
13. Akakura K, Bruchovsky N, Goldenberg SL et al (1993) Effects of intermittent androgen suppression on androgen-dependent tumors. Apoptosis and serum prostate specific antigen. Cancer 71:2782–2790
14. Gleave M, Bruchovsky N, Goldenberg SL et al (1998) Intermittent androgen suppression for prostate cancer: rationale and clinical experience. Eur Urol 34(Suppl 3):37S–41S
15. Klotz LH, Herr HW, Morse MJ et al (1986) Intermittent endocrine therapy for advanced prostate cancer. Cancer 58:2546–2550
16. Tunn U (2008) Can intermittent hormone therapy fulfil its promise? Eur Urol Suppl 7:752–757
17. Tunn U (2007) The current status of intermittent androgen deprivation (IAD) therapy for prostate cancer: putting IAD under the spotlight. BJU Int 99(Suppl 1):19–22
18. Gleave M, Klotz L, Taneja SS (2009) The continued debate: intermittent vs. continuous hormonal ablation for metastatic prostate cancer. Urol Oncol 27:81–86
19. Shaw G, Oliver RTD (2009) Intermittent hormone therapy and its place in the contemporary endocrine treatment of prostate cancer. Surg Oncol 18:275–282
20. Boccon-Gibod L, Hammerer P, Madersbacher S et al (2007) The role of intermittent androgen deprivation in prostate cancer. BJU Int 100:738–743
21. Shaw GL, Wilson P, Cuzick J et al (2007) International study into the use of intermittent hormone therapy in the treatment of carcinoma of the prostate: a meta-analysis of 1446 patients. BJU Int 99:1056–1065
22. Abrahamsson PA (2010) Potential benefits of intermittent androgen suppression therapy in the treatment of prostate cancer: a systematic review of the literature. Eur Urol 57:49–59
23. Bruchovsky N, Klotz L, Crook J et al (2007) Locally advanced prostate cancer—biochemical results from a prospective phase II study of intermittent androgen suppression for men with evidence of prostate-specific antigen recurrence after radiotherapy. Cancer 109:858–867

24. Bruchovsky N, Klotz L, Crook J et al (2008) Quality of life, morbidity, and mortality results of a prospective phase II study of intermittent androgen suppression for men with evidence of prostate-specific antigen relapse after radiation therapy for locally advanced prostate cancer. Clin Genitourin Cancer 6:46–52
25. Bruchovsky N, Klotz L, Crook J et al (2006) Final results of the Canadian prospective phase II trial of intermittent androgen suppression for men in biochemical recurrence after radiotherapy for locally advanced prostate cancer: clinical parameters. Cancer 107:389–395
26. Strum SB, Scholz MC, McDermed JE (2000) Intermittent androgen deprivation in prostate cancer patients: factors predictive of prolonged time off therapy. Oncologist 5:45–52
27. Leibowitz RL, Tucker SJ (2001) Treatment of localized prostate cancer with intermittent triple androgen blockade: preliminary results in 110 consecutive patients. Oncologist 6:177–182
28. Mottet N, Van Damme J, Loulidi S et al (2012) TAP22 Investigators Group. Intermittent hormone therapy in the treatment of metastatic prostate cancer: a randomized trial. BJU Int 110:1262–1269
29. Crook JM, O'Calleghan C, Dincan G et al (2012) Intermittent androgen suppression for rising PSA level after radiotherapy [published correction appears in N Engl J Med 2012;367:2262]. N Engl J Med 367:895–903
30. Hussain M, Tangen CM, Berry DL et al (2013) Intermittent versus continuous androgen deprivation in prostate cancer. N Engl J Med 368:1314–1325
31. De Leval J, Boca P, Yousef E (2002) Intermittent versus continuous total androgen blockade in the treatment of patients with advanced hormone-naïve prostate cancer: results of a prospective randomize multicentre trial. Clin Prostate Cancer 1:163–171
32. Langenhuijsen JF, Badhauser D, Schaaf B et al (2013) Continuous versus intermittent androgen deprivation therapy for metastatic prostate cancer. Urol Oncol 31(5):549–556
33. Calais da Silva F, Bono A, Whelan P et al (2009) Intermittent androgen deprivation for locally advanced and metastatic prostate cancer: results from a randomized phase 3 study of the South European Uroncological Group. Eur Urol 52:1269–1277
34. Salonen AJ, Taari K, Ala-Opas M, FinnProstate Group et al (2012) The FinnProstate Study VII: intermittent versus continuous androgen deprivation in patients with advanced prostate cancer. J Urol 187:2074–2081
35. Tunn U, Eckhart O, Kienle E et al (2003) Intermittent androgen deprivation in patients with PSA relapse after radical prostatectomy - first results of a randomised prospective phase-III clinical trial (AUO study AP06/95). Eur Urol Suppl 2(1):24
36. Gruca D, Bacher P, Tunn U (2012) Safety and tolerability of intermittent androgen deprivation therapy: a literature review. Int J Urol 19:614–625
37. Silva FC, Silva FM, Goncalves F et al (2013) Locally advanced and metastatic prostate cancer treated with intermittent androgen monotherapy or maximal androgen blockade: results from a randomised phase 3 study by the South European Uroncological Group. Eur Urol. doi:10.1016/j.eururo.2013.03.055
38. Conti PD, Atallah AN, Arruda H et al (2007) Intermittent versus continuous androgen suppression for prostate cancer. Cochrane Database Syst Rev CD005009
39. Prapotnich D, Fizazi K, Escudier B et al (2003) A 10-year clinical experience with intermittent hormonal therapy for prostate cancer. Eur Urol 43:233–240, discussion 239–240
40. Scholz MC, Lam RY, Strum SB et al (2011) Primary intermittent androgen deprivation as initial therapy for men with newly diagnosed prostate cancer. Clin Genitourin Cancer 9(2):89–94
41. Shore N, Crawford D (2010) Intermittent androgen deprivation therapy: redefining the standard of care? Rev Urol 12:1–11
42. Benaim EA, Pace CM, Lam PM et al (2002) Nadir prostate specific antigen as a predictor of progression to androgen independent prostate cancer. Urology 59(1):73–78
43. Sciarra A, Cattarino S, Gentilucci A et al (2013) Predictors for response to intermittent androgen deprivation (IAD) in prostate cancer cases with biochemical progression after surgery. Urol Oncol 31(5):607–614. doi:10.1016/j.urolonc.2011.05.005

44. Yu EY, Gulati R, Telesca D et al (2010) Duration of first off-treatment interval is prognostic for time to castration resistance and death in men with biochemical relapse of prostate cancer treated on a prospective trial of intermittent androgen deprivation. J Clin Oncol 28(16):2668–2673
45. Morote J, Orsola A, Planas J et al (2007) Redefining clinically significant castration levels in patients with prostate cancer receiving continuous androgen deprivation therapy. J Urol 178 (4):1290–1295
46. Spry NA, Galvão DA, Davies R et al (2009) Long-term effects of intermittent androgen suppression on testosterone recovery and bone mineral density: results of a 33-month observational study. BJU Int 104(6):806–812
47. Niraula S, Le LW, Tannock IF (2013) Treatment of prostate cancer with intermittent versus continuous androgen deprivation: a systematic review of randomized trials. J Clin Oncol 31 (16):2029–2036

Flavia Longo

10.1 Introduction

Androgen-deprivation therapy (ADT) is the standard treatment for advanced and metastatic prostate adenocarcinoma [1]. However, ADT resistance will eventually develop therefore leading into a poor clinical outcome [2] with a median survival (OS) of 16–18 months if no further treatment is administered [3]. Adding a first-generation antiandrogen such as flutamide, bicalutamide, or nilutamide to attain, a combined androgen blockade (CAB) can result in PSA response but usually this is short-living and no real improvement in OS has been demonstrated [4]. In the long term, a first-generation peripheral antiandrogen can induce paradoxal stimulation of the androgen receptor; therefore, discontinuation of these drugs is recommended. A further hormone manipulation in the form of the antifungal ketoconazole has demonstrated to be effective in reducing PSA; however, the short duration of response as well as the toxicities associated would preclude recommendation for this drug [4]. However, the continuing expression of PSA [5], an androgen receptor (AR)-regulated gene, clearly demonstrates that the AR pathway is still active at molecular level. Hence, the speculation that prostate cancer is not "androgen independent," but "castration resistant" instead [1, 6, 7].

F. Longo (✉)
Department of Medical Oncology, University Sapienza Rome, Viale del Policlinico 155, Rome 00144, Italy
e-mail: Flavia.longo@uniroma1.it

10.2   Molecular Biology

10.2.1 Mechanisms of Resistance

There are many models proposed to explain the prostate cancer transition into a castration-resistant status and it has been shown that numerous and not mutually exclusive factors are involved in this progression.

An interesting model has been proposed by Logothetis et al. who describe a three successive phase process in prostate cancer progression, namely endocrine-driven, microenvironment-dependent, and tumor cell autonomous [8]. Androgen signaling plays a pivotal role in this model of tumor progression. In the early first phase, androgen signaling responds to dihydrotestosterone (DHT) depletion—a vast proportion of low-grade and early-stage prostate cancers are in this "DHT-dependent" stage at diagnosis; however, upon escaping DHT dependence, cancers are characterized by paracrine-driven progression. This transition is a landmark of entry into a vicious circle where numerous changes in androgen signaling are associated with an aberrant microenvironment/tumor interaction. In the last phase of disease, cancer cells lose AR dependence, therefore exiting this paracrine progression spiral and becoming tumor cell autonomous (Fig. 10.1). In vitro studies have demonstrated that prostate cancer cells surviving androgen-depleted conditions eventually express increased levels of stem cell markers and are able to repopulate the tumor, through AR pathway adaptation [9].

According to this model, the transition from endocrine to paracrine-driven prostate cancer is associated with a number of modifications involving both oncogenes activation and tumor suppressor genes loss (e.g., loss of the PTEN tumor suppressor protein leads to uncontrolled activity of the phosphoinositide 3-kinase (PI3K)/Akt pathway). During the microenvironment-dependent phase, cancer progression is dominated by tumor adaptive changes and these modifications will end up in a vicious circle, in which the microenvironment alters the tumors and the tumor in turn modify the microenvironment. Emerging evidences suggest that there is a bidirectional crosstalk between several oncogenes and AR; therefore, activation of oncogenes and androgen depletion are not independent functions [8]. Among main changes we can identify the following:

Upregulation of enzymes involved in steroidogenesis—particularly intratumoral steroidogenesis and in the adrenal glands.

AR gene amplifications that lead to an AR overexpression and therefore possibly a hypersensitivity to androgen ligands. Castration-resistant patients with AR amplification respond at a higher rate to second-line maximal androgen blockade when compared to those without amplification [10].

   Although castration, the hypersensitivity of AR to low levels of androgens results in a continuous tumor growth.

   Prostate cancer (PC) xenograft models demonstrate how an increased expression of AR is the main aberration found in ADT refractory tumors and a high level of AR is overexpressed in CRPC tumors [2].

AR mutations: the AR gene is the most mutated type of steroid receptor. Most of the AR mutations are gain-of-function mutations. These can be mapped on the ligand-binding domain and eventually will result into androgen hypersensitivity

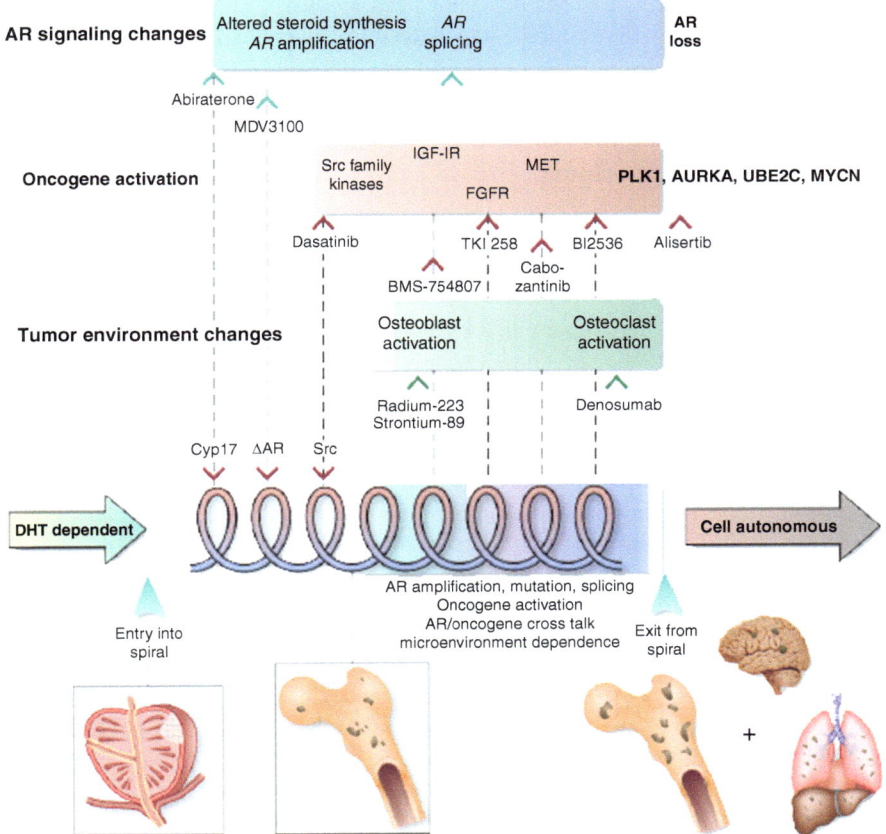

Fig. 10.1 Proposed spiral model for prostate cancer progression by Logothetis [8]

or AR decreased ligand specificity. More than 660 AR mutations have been reported thus far [11]. The presence of mutation of AR in Caucasians with an untreated localized PCa is <2 %, but the frequency of AR mutations may vary ranging between 20 and 50 % in metastatic castration-resistant tumors. These mutations may involve false triggering from other steroid hormones. These mutations allow AR to be activated by noncanonical ligands, like other steroids [2] or from treatments initially used as antiandrogens. The latter phenomenon is known as "antagonist-to-agonist" conversion and explains the "antiandrogen withdrawal" effect, i.e., the decline in PSA manifested in ~25 % of patients following the discontinuation of these drugs after clinical progression [1, 12, 13]. *Epigenetic modifications* such as methylation of the AR receptor and AR *splicing variant* in promoting a constitutive gene expression. The *role of co-activators and co-repressors* in the development of castration-resistant disease is still not completely clear and so is it the role of AR *post-translational modifications*

(PTMs). Most of the PTMs have not been studied within the in vivo human context and they will need to be translated into clinical experience to understand clinical utility [14].

10.2.2 Clinical Experience

10.2.2.1 Role of Taxanes in CRPC

Docetaxel-based chemotherapy is the established standard of care at development of castration-resistant prostate cancer. This drug was proven to be superior to the previous standard of care represented by mitoxantrone. The latter was assessed in a randomized phase III trial in which patients were randomized to mitoxantrone and corticosteroids vs. single use of steroids. Mitoxantrone in improvement of pain, QoL, and PSA response, but overall survival (OS) was similar [15, 16]. The first trial showing superiority of docetaxel over mitoxantrone was the SWOG 99-16, in which the combination of docetaxel and estramustine was demonstrated to be superior to mitoxantrone and prednisone [17, 18]. However, the main phase III trial which led to registration of docetaxel as standard of care for progressing CRPC was the TAX327; in this trial, 1,006 men with metastatic CRPC received 5 mg of prednisone twice daily and were randomly assigned to receive ten courses of 3-weekly mitoxantrone or weekly (5 weeks out of 6) docetaxel or 3-weekly docetaxel, respectively. The study proved that 3-weekly docetaxel and prednisone was the preferred treatment leading to an improvement of overall survival and quality of life with a better pain control and a better biochemical response [19]. According to this trial, docetaxel given every 3 weeks has become the standard of care in symptomatic CPRC patients.

Apart from a direct cytotoxic activity, there is increasing interest and at least in vitro evidence of an "antihormonal" mechanism of action of docetaxel and taxanes in general [20]. Decreased expression of AR-transactivated genes through the inhibition of AR transcriptional activity represents a new potential molecular pathway that could explain efficacy of taxanes in the treatment of prostate cancer [21].

Cabazitaxel (JEVTANA®)

Cabazitaxel was the first demonstrated drug to improve survival in patients with CRPC progressing after treatment with docetaxel. This drug is a member of the taxane family, which includes paclitaxel and docetaxel. Cabazitaxel binds to tubulin and promotes assembly into microtubules and inhibits disassembly, resulting in stabilization of microtubules, which interferes with mitotic and cellular interphase activity [22]. It shows a power comparable to that of docetaxel in cellular line but the uniqueness of having antitumor activity in models resistant to paclitaxel and docetaxel [23–25], and also the ability to cross the blood–brain barrier.

The study that led to the approval by the FDA of cabazitaxel was the TROPIC, an open-label randomized phase III trial in men with metastatic castration-resistant prostate cancer who had received previous hormone therapy, but whose disease had progressed during or after treatment with a docetaxel-containing regimen.

In this study, 755 patients were enrolled, 378 received cabazitaxel 25 mg/m^2 intravenously over 1 h and oral prednisone 10 mg daily. Patients under treatment with LHRH agonists and bisphosphonates continued treatment along the study.

Eligible patients were aged at least 18 years, with an Eastern Cooperative Oncology Group (ECOG) PS 0–2. Patients who had previous mitoxantrone therapy, radiotherapy to 40 % or more of the bone marrow, or cancer therapy (other LHRH analogues) within 4 weeks before enrollment were excluded. Patients with measurable disease were required to have disease progression with at least one visceral or soft-tissue metastatic lesion. Patients with nonmeasurable disease were required to have rising PSA in two consecutive measurements or at least one new demonstrable radiographic lesion before enrollment; adequate hematological, hepatic, renal, and cardiac function, and a left-ventricular ejection fraction $\geq$50 % assessed by multigated radionuclide angiography or echocardiogram.

Results proved that median survival in people taking cabazitaxel was 15.1 months vs. 12.7 months in the mitoxantrone group. The hazard ratio for death of men treated with cabazitaxel compared with those taking mitoxantrone was 0.70 (95 % CI 0.59–0.83, $P < 0.0001$). The median progression-free survival was 2.8 months compared with 1.4 of mitoxantrone (HR 0.74, 0.64–0.86, $P < 0.0001$). Most significant adverse were neutropenia (cabazitaxel vs. mitoxantrone 83 58 %), diarrhea (6 % vs. 1 %), and febrile neutropenia (8 % vs. 1 %). The high incidence of febrile neutropenia suggests that treatment requires prophylaxis [26].

An update of the study to 25.5 months also shows more patients remained alive following cabazitaxel than mitoxantrone [odds ratio 2.11; 95 % confidence interval (CI) 1.33–3.33]. Treatment with cabazitaxel was prognostic for survival $\geq$2 years; in fact, the probability of surviving $\geq$2 years was 27 % (95 % CI 23–32 %) with cabazitaxel vs. 16 % (95 % CI 12–20 %) with mitoxantrone. Pain at baseline and pain response were comparable between treatment groups. Average daily pain performance index was lower for cabazitaxel vs. mitoxantrone (all cycles; 95 % CI −0.27 to −0.01; $P = 0.035$) and analgesic scores were similar. Grade $\geq$3 peripheral neuropathies were uncommon and comparable between treatment groups [27].

A phase III clinical trial comparing the efficacy and toxicity of cabazitaxel 20 mg/m^2 prednisone vs. cabazitaxel 25 mg/m^2 (PROSELICA; NCT01308580) is ongoing [28].

Cabazitaxel is also being evaluated in a first-line phase III trial (FIRSTANA; NCT01308567). In this open-label trial, 1,170 patients with chemotherapy-naïve mCRPC will be randomized to docetaxel (75 mg/m^2 every 3 weeks) or cabazitaxel (20 or 25 mg/m^2 every 3 weeks) plus prednisone (10 mg orally, daily) [29].

10.2.2.2 CYP17 Inhibitors
Abiraterone (Zytiga®)
Abiraterone acetate is new potent hormonotherapy recently developed and approved for treatment of CRPC. This drug represents the "proof-of-concept" that prostate cancer remains hormone driven even after failure of androgen deprivation therapy. The reason of developing such a drug started off from the observation that patients exposed to ketoconazole—a known antifungal treatment essentially able to inhibit the CYP17 enzyme which is key in male sex hormones production—could achieve some

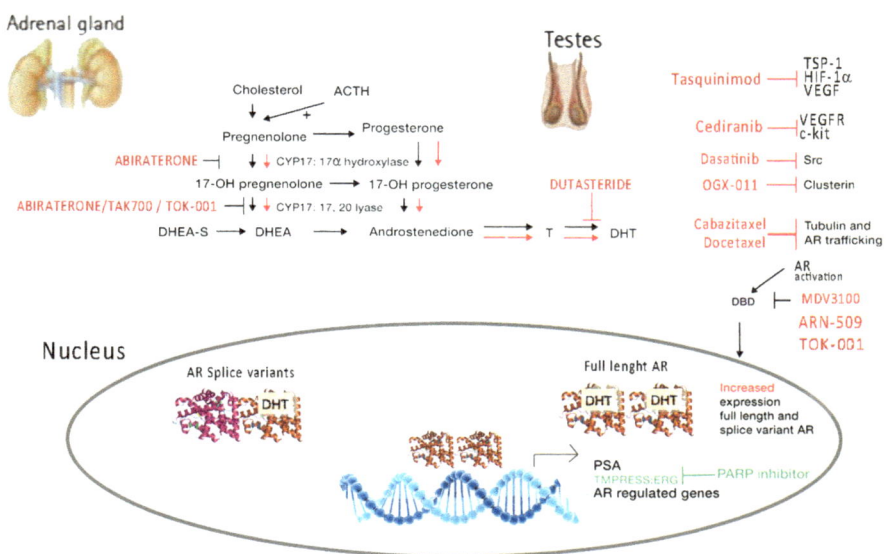

Fig. 10.2 Mechanism of action of new drugs in the treatment of CRPC

response at least in terms of PSA drop because of its ability to prevent prostate cancer cells growth. However, ketoconazole is poorly tolerated and its affinity for CYP17 is low. Research conducted at the Institute of cancer Research UK led to the development of a potent CYP17 inhibitor, which was called CB7598 or abiraterone. However, this drug raised the question of the potential-related side effects, namely the risk of causing adrenal insufficiency. However, the clinical observation that children born with a deficiency of the CYP17 enzyme did not develop adrenal insufficiency (http://www.icr.ac.uk/press/recent_featured_articles/Story_Abiraterone/index.shtml), led to the initial clinical application of the drug (Fig. 10.2).

The phase I and II trials carried out in men with castration-resistant prostate cancer showed that the drug was very well tolerated with no major side effects and also some interesting preliminary efficacy in terms substantial PSA decline. Radiological response was also reported with evidence of partial responses in patients with measurable disease [30]. The phase III international, randomized, double-blind, placebo-controlled trial called COU-AA-301 finally led to the approval of abiraterone acetate in castration-resistant prostate cancer patients previously exposed to docetaxel. In this trial, 1,195 patients received prednisolone and 1 g of abiraterone acetate or placebo on a fasted status daily. Treatment could be continued until PSA, radiological and clinical disease progression was documented. Results of the final results analysis—updated in 2012—show that group taking abiraterone of 15.8 months compared to 11.2 months in the group taking placebo (hazard ratio [HR] 0.74, 95 % CI 0.64–0.86, $P < 0.0001$). Median time to PSA progression was 8.5 months for the group treated with abiraterone vs. 6.6 months (HR 0.63, 0.52–0.78, $P < 0.0001$), similar to the median radiologic progression-free survival (5.6 months vs. 3.6 months, HR 0.66, 12:58–0.76, $P < 0.0001$). PSA responses (29.5 % vs. 5.5 %, $P < 0.0001$) were all improved in the abiraterone group compared with placebo group. Adverse events grade 3–4 related to the use of abiraterone were: fatigue, anemia, back pain, and bone pain [31]. The approval from the U.S. Food and Drug Administration (FDA) for hormone refractory prostate cancer, in post-docetaxel setting, was given in April 2011 and the European approval was followed in September 2011. More recently, abiraterone has been investigated in asymptomatic or paucisymptomatic patients with CRPC before administration of docetaxel. Based on experiences of previous earlier phase of development trials [32–34], investigated the potential use of abiraterone acetate in 1,088 castration-resistant patients not previously treated with docetaxel were randomized to receive prednisone and abiraterone or placebo in phase III international, double-blind, placebo-controlled study. The results from an interim analysis showed that the median radiographic progression-free survival (PFS) was 16.5 months with the use of abiraterone–prednisone and 8.3 months with only prednisone (HR, 0.53; 95 % [CI], 0.45–0.62, $P < 0.001$). However, on a follow-up of 22.2 months, the primary end point of the trial overall survival (OS) was not met as there were not enough related events in the abiraterone arm (vs. 27.2 months for prednisone alone, HR 0.75, 95 % CI, 0.61–0.93, $P = 0.01$). The drug also demonstrated superiority over placebo, for opiate use for cancer-related pain, prostate-specific antigen progression, and decline in performance status [35]. Nevertheless, based on these results abiraterone acetate was approved by FDA in the predocetaxel setting in December 2012. In keeping with its clinical efficacy, abiraterone is able to affect the detection of circulating tumor cells with the Cell Search machine and results seem to correlate closely with overall survival of patients. Studies are ongoing to assess the efficacy of abiraterone in combination with LHRH analogues is hormonotherapy naïve patients (NCT01088529 and NCT00924469) as well as pre and concomitant to radical radiotherapy (NCT01023061). Eventually, patients exposed to abiraterone acetate will develop resistance to this therapy; therefore, the basic and clinical research is aiming to understand mechanism and develop strategies to overcome that. Combination treatments with chemotherapy [36] or other agents, such as PI3K (phosphoinositide 3-kinase)/AKT (a serine/threonine protein kinase) inhibitors and PARP inhibitors [37], are ongoing and results from clinical experience are awaited [38].

TOK-001 (Galeterone)
Galeterone (also known as TOK-001) was rationally designed to inhibit the human CYP17 enzyme, but was also found to be a potent pure AR antagonist and to effectively prevent the binding of synthetic androgens to both mutant and wild-type AR [39, 40] (Fig. 10.2). A phase I, multicentre, dose-finding study in patients with chemotherapy naïve CRPC was published in the American Society of Clinical Oncology (ASCO) meeting in 2012. Patients were enrolled in cohorts from 650 to 2,600 mg of TOK-001 daily, with 36 of 49 completing the 12-week treatment course. The treatment was generally well tolerated, with only one severe AE considered related to TOK-001 (rhabdomyolysis with acute renal failure, with

high-dose statin use). Overall 22 % of treated patients had a >50 % PSA level decline, and an additional 26 % had 30–50 % PSA level declines. Consistent with lyase inhibition, increased corticosteroids, and suppressed androgens were seen with dose escalation [41].

Tak-700 (Ortonel)

TAK-700 selectively inhibits the CYP17A 17, 20 lyase [42], whose task is to reduce in vivo levels of androgens produced by the adrenal gland (Fig. 10.2). Dreicer et al, tested tak-700 in a phase I/II open-label, dose-escalation to test safety in 26 mCRPC patients of oral twice daily (BID) TAK-700. All patients treated with ≥300 mg had a PSA decrease, of 15 patients who received TAK-700 ≥ 300 mg for ≥3 cycles and had a 3-month PSA determination, 12 (80 %) had ≥50 % PSA reductions and 4 (27 %) had ≥90 % reductions. Median testosterone and DHEA sulfate levels decreased from 5.5 to 0.6 ng/dL and from 50.0 µg/dL [43].

10.2.2.3 AR Antagonists
Enzalutamide (Xtandi®)

Enzalutamide (formerly MDV3100) is an androgen receptor signaling inhibitor chosen for clinical development on the basis of activity in prostate-cancer models with overexpression of the androgen receptor. Enzalutamide is distinct from the currently available antiandrogen agents that inhibit nuclear translocation of androgen receptor, DNA binding, and coactivator recruitment. It also has a greater affinity for the receptor, induces tumor shrinkage in xenograft models (conventional agents only retard growth), and has no known agonistic effects [13, 44] (Fig. 10.2).

Enzalutamide has been approved by the FDA in July 2012 for CRPC patients, following docetaxel chemotherapy.

Enzalutamide is administered once daily, without the need for concomitant prednisone which has been postulated to activate androgen receptor signaling.

One of the first studies of Scher's team showed that in a population of 140 subjects there was at least a PSA halving in 56 % of patients, soft tissue response in 22 %, stable bone disease in 56 %, and a reduction below threshold levels of circulating tumor cells in 49 %; moreover, there was a median time to radiological progression of 47 weeks. Among adverse effects of grade 3–4 11 % complained fatigue usually resolved with dose reduction. So results proved that MDV3100 has a substantial antitumor activity in men with castration-resistant prostate cancer, whether or not they have been exposed to chemotherapy [5].

The potential of the drug has been confirmed by analysis of the AFFIRM group (A Study Evaluating the Efficacy and Safety of the Investigational Drug MDV3100) that enlists 1,199 subjects in a phase III, double-blind, placebo-controlled trial. Among inclusion criteria of the study were presence of testosterone levels <50 ng/dL [1.7 nmol/L], previous treatment with docetaxel and progressive disease defined according to Functional PCWG2 criteria. The use of prednisone or other glucocorticoids was allowed but not required. Important to note that patients were maintained on GnRH agonist/antagonist therapy and could receive supportive care medications.

The median overall survival was 18.4 months in the group treated with the enzalutamide respect to 13.6 months in the placebo group (hazard ratio for death in the enzalutamide group, 0.63, 95 % CI, 0.75–0.53, $P < 0.001$). The enzalutamide declared itself superior over placebo in all secondary end points: the proportion of patients with a reduction in the prostate-specific antigen (PSA) level by 50 % or more (54 % vs. 2 %, $P < 0.001$), the soft-tissue response rate (29 % vs. 4 %, $P < 0.001$), the quality-of-life response rate (43 % vs. 18 %, $P < 0.001$), the time to PSA progression (8.3 vs. 3.0 months, hazard ratio, 0.25, $P < 0.001$), radiographic progression-free survival (8.3 vs. 2.9 months, hazard ratio, 0.40; $P < 0.001$), and the time to the first skeletal-related event (16.7 vs. 13.3 months, hazard ratio 0.69, $P < 0.001$).

Among the major adverse events related to the use of MDV3100 stands fatigue, lightheadedness, and hot flushes. It is appropriate to specify how the average time from onset of any adverse event of grade 3 or higher was 8.4 months longer in the group that took enzalutamide than placebo group (12.6 vs. 4.2 months), so leading to an improvement in long-term control of disease without an increase of the reactions events.

Should also be noted that in 0.6 % of the population examined occurred seizures, in some cases in people with predisposing conditions or concomitant treatments: physicians should pay particular attention when administering enzalutamide in patients with a history of epilepsy or with predisposing factors (underlying brain injury, stroke, brain metastases, alcoholism, or patients taking drugs that lower the seizure threshold) [18].

In order to better understand the potential use of the drug is now ongoing a phase III trial in chemo-naïve patients (PREVAIL; NCT01212991).

ARN-509

ARN-509 is a drug able to inhibit AR nuclear translocation, AR binding to androgen response elements and, unlike bicalutamide, does not exhibit agonist properties in the context of AR overexpression (Fig. 10.2). In its first inhuman phase I study, PSA declines at 12 weeks (≥ 50 % reduction from baseline) were observed in 46.7 % of patients. Reduction in FDHT uptake was present at all doses, with a plateau in response at ≥ 120-mg dose, consistent with saturation of AR binding. Assessed in this study were also safety, tolerability, pharmacokinetics, pharmacodynamics, and antitumor activity of ARN-509 in men with metastatic CRPC [45].

10.2.2.4 Immunotherapy
Sipuleucel-T (Provenge®)

Immunotherapy is emerging as a therapeutic strategy for patients with prostate cancer. There are numerous strategies approachable in the use of the immune system and between them stands the production of cancer vaccines designed to stimulate the immune cells against target expressed by cancer cells.

Sipuleucel-T (APC8015) is an autologous active cellular immunotherapy used in the treatment of men with asymptomatic or minimally symptomatic metastatic castration-resistant prostate cancer (CRPC). It is the first therapeutic cancer vaccine to receive U.S. FDA approval. Sipuleucel-T is an "active cellular immunotherapy," a type of cancer vaccine consisting of autologous peripheral blood mononuclear cells (PBMCs), including antigen-presenting cells (APCs), which were activated ex vivo with a recombinant fusion protein (PA2024). The APCs are then incubated with a recombinant protein composed of prostatic acid phosphatase (PAP) linked to granulocyte-macrophage colony-stimulating factor (GM-CSF) [46]. PAP was chosen as the target antigen because is expressed in prostate tissues and in the vast majority of carcinomas of the prostate with a no or minimal expression in other tissues [47], also does not share a high degree of sequence homology with any other protein know. Task of GM-CSF is instead to increase the uptake of APCs [48].

Approximately 3 days prior to each infusion of sipuleucel-T, patients undergo a leukapheresis procedure for collection of autologous peripheral blood mononuclear cells. Preparation of sipuleucel-T Involves enrichment for antigen-presenting cells from the leukapheresis product and activation ex vivo with a recombinant fusion protein (PA2024).

As early as 2006, the randomized, placebo-controlled study of Small and colleagues showed how, by analyzing 127 patients, the median time to disease progression (TTP) for sipuleucel-T was 11.7 weeks compared with 10.0 weeks for placebo ($P = 0.052$, log-rank; hazard ratio [HR], 1.45; 95 % CI, 0.99–2.11). Survival rate at 3 years was stated to 34.1 %, with an average increase of 4.5 months and a median survival of 25.9 months. The treatment was also well tolerated by patients. It is important to note, however, as the primary end point (TTP) has not been reached [49].

A second study of 225 patients from the group of Higano showed a trend of increase in survival with sipuleucel-T despite not statistically significant. There was also an insignificant effect on time to disease progression (PFS) [50].

Fundamental to approve the sipuleucel-T was the phase III study called Immunotherapy for Prostate adenocarcinoma Treatment (IMPACT). Structured as a double-blind, placebo-controlled, multicenter trial enrolled patients with any Gleason score, asymptomatic or minimally symptomatic, PSA $\geq$ 5 ng/mL, serum testosterone $<$ 50 ng/dL (17 nmol/L). Exclusion criteria included a baseline ECOG PS greater ≥ 2, presence of visceral metastases, pathological fractures of long bones, compression of the spinal cord, within 28 days of treatment with glucocorticoids, prior external beam radiation, surgery, or systemic treatment for cancer prostate (except for medical or surgical castration). Exclusion criteria include also the use of bisphosphonates in previous 28 days, history of treatment with two or more chemotherapy regimens, or chemotherapy within 3 months. The continuation of chemical castration or bisphosphonate therapy has been requested at least until the time of disease progression.

All 512 patients were randomly assigned in a 2:1 ratio to receive sipuleucel-T or placebo every 2 weeks for three infusions. Subjects enrolled had received prior androgen deprivation. Be mentioned that the average age was 71 years.

Results of the analysis proved as in the group with sipuleucel-T the adjusted hazard ratio for death was 0.78 (95 % CI, 0.61–0.98) and that reduction in the risk of death was 22 % ($P = 0.03$). The median survival of 4.1 months stood higher than the control group (25.8 months vs. 21.7 months). The probability of survival at 36 months was 31.7 % in the group taking sipuleucel-T and 23.0 % in the placebo group.

The median time to progression disease was 14.6 weeks (3.7 months) in the group treated with sipuleucel-T and 14.4 weeks (3.6 months) in the placebo group (hazard ratio 0.92, 95 % CI, 0.75–1.12, $P = 0:40$). Among patients with periodic evaluations of PSA, a reduction of at least 50 % was observed in 8 of 311 patients (2.6 %) in subjects treated with sipuleucel-T compared to 1.3 % of the control group (2 of 152 patients).

Among the major adverse effects experienced in the group taking sipuleucel-T was found were chills, fever (pyrexia), headache, flu-like illness, myalgia, hypertension, hyperhidrosis, and groin pain. Except for groin pain, most of these events have occurred the day following the infusion and resolved within 1 or 2 days. Overall, only 3 of 338 patients (0.9 %) in the group sipuleucel-T were not able to receive all three infusions because of adverse events related to the infusion [51].

Due to these results in April 2010, the Food and Drug Administration (FDA) has authorized sipuleucel-T in the treatment of metastatic castration-resistant disease in patients asymptomatic or minimally symptomatic.

Although there are no short-term changes in disease progression or available biomarkers to assess response, these agents appear to improve survival. One hypothesis suggests that this apparent paradox can be explained by the growth-moderating effects of treatments, which do not cause tumor size to diminish, but rather stall or slow their growth rate over time [52]. For this reason, further studies should clarify the real benefits in relation to other treatments.

PROSTVAC (TRICOM®)

In development is also PROSTVAC a fowlpox vaccines and vectors with a triade of costimulatory molecule transgenes, including intercellular adhesion molecule 1 (ICAM-1), B7.1, and leukocyte function-associated antigen 3 (LFA-3), which has been designated TRICOM® [53]. In a randomized double-blind phase II trial, patients with a mild or asymptomatic metastatic chemo-naive PCa, Gleason score ≤7 and rising PSA were randomized to receive placebo or PROSTVAC. Patients on the vaccine arm achieved an improved median survival of 24.5 months compared with 16 months in the placebo group $P = 0.016$ [54]. T-cell activation is dependent on two separate signals: the first is the presentation of an antigen linked to the major histocompatibility complex (MHC) molecule and the second is a costimulatory of the interaction of CD28 on the T cell with CD80 and CD86 on the APC. Both CD28 and cytotoxic T lymphocyte-associated antigen 4 (CTLA-4) are expressed on T cells, and competitively bind to the same ligands present on APCs. In contrast to the activating function of CD28 however, CTLA-4 serves as an immunomodulatory molecule that negatively regulates T-cell activation and dampens the immune response generated. This inhibitory feedback is integral for the maintenance of peripheral tolerance of self-antigens and can be exploited therapeutically by targeting CTLA-4 to enhance T-cell-mediated antitumor immune responses.

Similarly, PROVASTAC VF showed a statistically significant survival difference of 8.5 months (25.1 vs. 16.6 months, estimated 0.56 HR 95 % CI, 0.85–12:37; stratified log-rank $P = 0.0061$) in a randomized, placebo-controlled trial [55]. Another single-arm phase II trial of PROSTVAC in mCRPC patients proved similar survival outcomes, with a median OS of 26.6 months [56]. A phase II trial randomized 26 patients with nonmetastatic CRPC to receive flutamide alone or with PROSTVAC-V/F reported preliminary that patients in the combination arm had improved time to progression compared with patients who received flutamide alone (223 vs. 85 days, respectively) [57].

Ipilimumab (Yervoy®)

Ipilimumab is a humanized monoclonal antibody against cytotoxic T lymphocyte antigen-4 (CTLA-4). CTLA-4, a T-cell surface receptor, is a key negative regulator of T-cell responses. Thus, ipilimumab augments antitumor immune response by inhibiting a negative regulator of T cells. Showing useful in some phase II studies with both castration [58] and PSA-TRICOM [59], serious difficulties were in the phase III trial CA-184-043 trial (Study 043) that enrolled 799 patients with mCRPC who had received prior docetaxel. In this trial, patients were randomized in a 1:1 ratio to receive bone-directed radiation therapy at 8 Gy followed by ipilimumab at 10 mg/kg ($n = 399$) or placebo ($n = 400$). A subgroup analysis suggests that patients with less advanced disease could still benefit from treatment with ipilimumab. The study failed to meet its primary end point of prolongation in overall survival (OS). Despite the lack of an OS benefit, progression-free survival (PFS) and a marked reduction in PSA were observed with immunotherapy.

Also, interesting is the trial by Madan et al. concerning ipilimumab in combination with a poxviral-based vaccine targeting prostate-specific antigen (PSA) and containing transgenes for T-cell costimulatory molecule expression, including CD80. Only one of the six patients previously treated with chemotherapy had a PSA decline from baseline. Of the 24 patients who were chemotherapy-naive, 14 (58 %) had PSA declines from baseline, of which six were greater than 50 %. The use of a vaccine targeting PSA that also enhances costimulation of the immune system did not seem to exacerbate the immune-related adverse events associated with ipilimumab [59]. Randomized trials are needed to further assess clinical outcomes of the combination of ipilimumab and vaccine in mCRPC.

10.2.2.5 Antiangiogenic Agents

Tasquinimod

Treatment with tasquinimod (TASQ) plays a role in the upregulation of TSP-1 expression and downregulation of HIF-1α and VEGF [60, 61] (Fig. 10.2). Preclinical data demonstrated that work synergistically with taxanes (docetaxel and cabazitaxel) [62, 63].

In a phase II trial by Pili et al., 201 patients were evaluated (134 assigned to TASQ; 67 to placebo). Six-month progression-free proportions for TASQ and placebo groups were 69 % and 37 %, respectively ($P < 0.001$), and median progression-free survival (PFS) was 7.6 vs. 3.3 months ($P = 0.0042$). So, TASQ significantly slowed progression and improved PFS in patients with metastatic CRPC with an acceptable AE profile [63]. Definitive assessment of tasquinimod in CRPC clinical treatment is still required and results of an ongoing major phase III clinical trials are awaited.

10.2.2.6 Tyrosine Kinase Inhibitors
Dasatinib (Sprycel®)
Dasatinib is an inhibitor of numerous kinases: BCR-ABL, SRC family (SRC, LCK, YES, and FYN), c-KIT, EphA2, and PDGFRβ. It is involved in multiple signaling pathways in prostate cancer and promotes tumor cell proliferation, survival, migration, and the transition to androgen independence. In experiments, dasatinib seems able to reduce the proliferation of osteoclasts and the release of calcium [64] (Fig. 10.2).

Dasatinib was tested in 48 chemotherapy-naïve men: a lack of disease progression was observed in 21 (44 %) patients at week 12 and in 8 (17 %) at week 24. Urine N-telopeptide was reduced by ≥40 % from baseline in 22 (51 %) of 43 patients, and bone alkaline phosphatase was decreased in 26 (59 %) of 44 patients. Dasatinib was well tolerated, with only 6 patients (13 %) grade 3–4 adverse events with drug related and 3 (6 %) with grade 3 adverse events [65].

Another study analyzed the potential association with docetaxel, experiencing durable 50 % PSA declines occurred in 26 of 46 patients (57 %). Of 30 patients with measurable disease, 18 (60 %) had a partial response. Twenty-eight patients (61 %) received single-agent dasatinib after docetaxel discontinuation and had stabilization of disease for an additional 1–12 months [66].

Interesting results come from the phase III study READY: a multinational, randomized, double-blinded, placebo-controlled. In this study, the addition of dasatinib to standard-of-care chemotherapy in mCRPC patients did not improve OS (median, 21.5 vs. 21.2 months; hazard ratio [HR], 0.99; log-rank $P = 0.90$), PFS (median, 11.8 vs. 11.1 months; HR, 0.92), and also pain reduction (66.6 vs. 71.5 %). Anyway there was a modest reduction in the risk of time to first skeletal-related eve with dasatinib (median, not reached vs. 31.1 months; HR, 0.81 [95 % CI, 0.64–1.02]) [67].

Cabozantinib (Cometriq®)
Cabozantinib (XL184) is an orally bioavailable tyrosine kinase inhibitor with activity against MET and vascular endothelial growth factor receptor 2. A phase II randomized discontinuation trial included a cohort of men with mCRPC, 43 % of whom had been previously treated with docetaxel. Men received 100 mg of cabozantinib daily for 12 weeks, and those with stable disease were randomized to either cabozantinib or placebo. Although the objective response rate at 12 weeks was only 5 %, 75 % had stable disease. Median PFS was 23.9 weeks (95 % CI, 10.7–62.4 weeks) with cabozantinib and 5.9 weeks (95 % CI, 5.4–6.6 weeks) with placebo (hazard ratio, 0.12; $P < 0.001$). Improvements in bone scans were noted in

68 %, with partial resolution in 56 % and complete resolution in 12 %. On retrospective review, bone pain improved in 67 % of evaluable patients, with a decrease in narcotic use in 56 %. All patients experienced at least one adverse event, often resulting in drug interruption and dose reduction [68]. Phase III trials of cabozantinib in the post-docetaxel setting are ongoing (NCT01605227 and NCT01522443).

10.2.2.7 PARP Inhibitors

Poly(ADP-ribose) polymerase (PARP) is implicated in DNA repair and transcription regulation. The inhibition of poly(adenosine diphosphate [ADP]-ribose) polymerase (PARP) is a potential synthetic lethal therapeutic strategy for the treatment of cancers with specific DNA-repair defects, including those arising in carriers of a BRCA1 or BRCA2 mutation (Fig. 10.2).

Olaparib

The potentiality of Olaparib was first tested by Fong et al. in 60 patients: 22 were carriers of a BRCA1 or BRCA2 mutation and 1 had a strong family history of BRCA-associated cancer but declined to undergo mutational testing. Objective antitumor activity was reported only in mutation carriers, all of whom had ovarian, breast, or prostate cancer and had received multiple treatment regimens. Olaparib showed few adverse effects of conventional chemotherapy, inhibits PARP, and has antitumor activity in cancer associated with the BRCA1 or BRCA2 mutation [69].

Niraparib

Another interesting drug is niraparib (MK4827) an oral potent, selective PARP-1 and PARP-2 inhibitor that induces synthetic lethality in preclinical tumor models with loss of BRCA and PTEN function. In the study of Sandhu et al., 8 of 20 BRCA1 or BRCA2 mutation carriers (40 % [95 % CI 19–64]) with ovarian cancer had RECIST partial responses, as did two of four mutation carriers with breast cancer (50 % [7–93]). Antitumor activity was also reported in sporadic high-grade serous ovarian cancer, nonsmall-cell lung cancer, and prostate cancer and was also recorded no correlation between loss of PTEN expression or ETS rearrangements and measures of antitumor activity in patients with prostate cancer [70].

10.2.2.8 Antisense Oligonucleotide

OGX-011 (Custirsen)

CLU is a stress-induced, cytoprotective chaperone upregulated to inhibit cell death that confers broad-spectrum resistance by inhibiting protein aggregation and proteotoxic stress, cytochrome C release, and Bax and caspase activation. CLU is an attractive candidate for inhibition at the mRNA level. Custirsen, a second-generation antisense oligonucleotide (ASO), has high affinity for CLU RNA, with increased potency, and a prolonged tissue half-life compared with first-generation ASOs (Fig. 10.2). Custirsen potently suppresses CLU levels both in vitro and in vivo [71, 72]. In a phase II study, 82 men with mCRPC were randomized (1:1) to docetaxel and prednisone with or without OGX-011. Although there was no improvement in PSA response (the primary end point), OS (secondary end point) was improved in the OGX-011 arm (23.8 months vs. 16.9 months) [73]. Currently, two phase III trials are ongoing to confirm these results in combination with chemotherapy: one in the first-line setting (SYNERGY, testing docetaxel with or without custirsen, NCT01188187), the other in the second-line setting (AFFINITY, testing cabazitaxel with and without custirsen, NCT01578655). Interesting are findings from Lamoureux et al. indicating that Hsp90 inhibitor-induced activation of the heat shock response and CLU is attenuated by OGX-011, with synergistic effects on delaying CRPC progression [74].

OGX-427

OGX-427 is an antisense oligonucleotide inhibiting the expression of heat shock protein 27, a chaperone protein that complexes with the AR and enhances transactivation of AR-regulated genes. In a phase II trial the use of OGX-427 and prednisone vs. prednisone alone was compared, the PFS at 12 weeks was 71 % (95 % CI 0.440–0.897) in the OGX-427 group and 40 % (95 % CI 0.163–0.677) in the prednisone alone arm [75]. The Hoosier Oncology Group is conducting a phase II study with OGX-427 in men with mCRPC who experience PSA progression on abiraterone acetate (NCT01681433) [76].

HSP-90

HSP90 is a molecular chaperone involved in the stability of many client proteins including Akt and androgen receptor (AR). 17-Allylamino-17-demethoxy-geldanamycin (17-AAG) has been reported to inhibit tumor growth in various cancers; however, it induces tumor progression in the bone microenvironment.

Results of several studies show that today Heat shock protein 90 inhibition is not an always an efficient target: IPI-504 administered as a single agent had a minimal effect on the PSA level or tumor burden and was associated with unacceptable toxicity in several patients [77]. Similarly, 17-AAG did not show any activity with regard to PSA response. Due to insufficient PSA response, enrollment was stopped at the end of first stage per study design [78, 79]. In any case, inhibitors of Hsp90 are still in a development stage and there are many molecules yet to be tested.

EZN-4176

EZN-4176, an androgen receptor (AR) mRNA antagonist, is a Locked Nucleic Acid (LNA) oligonucleotide that specifically down-modulates AR mRNA. In vitro, EZN-4176 has been shown to down-modulate AR mRNA and protein and inhibit AR transcriptional activity and cell growth. AR is widely recognized as an important therapeutic target for the treatment of prostate cancer, as androgens are essential to prostate tumor growth and viability. In the first-in-human phase I study, 22 patients were enrolled and there were no objective soft tissue responses. PD studies did not document any knockdown of AR expression. To date, EZN-4176 has limited antitumor activity in CRPC at its MTD for weekly administration [80].

10.2.2.9 Other Agents
Radium 223 Dichloride (Xofigo®)

Radium-223 dichloride (formerly called Alpharadin) is the first alpha emitter to undergo phase III testing and receive approval for clinical use, acts independently of cell cycles, surface markers, and tumor types. The simplicity of the alpha emitter radium-223 lies in its winning combination of a convenient half-life (11.4 days) and its inherent bone-seeking and potent DNA-damaging properties. The concept of relative biologic effectiveness combines physical linear energy transfers with the radiobiologic effects of ionizing radiation in tissue to provide a medically relevant scale for comparing the potencies of various forms of ionizing radiation. The relative biologic effectiveness of alpha emitters, which is several times that of traditional X-rays (depending on the tissue type), is their most and least attractive feature. Alpha particles are efficient, and they cause cell damage with a single knockout as compared with gamma rays and beta particles. Such killing power is rendered unattractive if it is coupled with an unforgiving half-life [81]. Parker et al. have developed the study Alpharadin in Symptomatic Prostate Cancer Patients (ALSYMPCA) a phase III, double-blind, placebo-controlled study, that randomly assigned 921 patients who had received, were not eligible to receive, or declined docetaxel, in a 2:1 ratio, to receive six injections of radium-223 (at a dose of 50 kBq/kg of body weight intravenously) or matching placebo; one injection was administered every 4 weeks. In addition, all patients received the best standard of care. An updated analysis, when 528 deaths had occurred, was performed before crossover from placebo to radium-223. At the interim analysis, the median overall survival was 14.0 months in the radium-223 group and 11.2 months in the placebo group. Radium-223, as compared with placebo, was associated with a 30 % reduction in the risk of death (hazard ratio, 0.70; 95 % confidence interval [CI], 0.55–0.88; two-sided $P = 0.002$). In the intention-to-treat population, 314 patients died. In the radium-223 group, 191 of 541 patients died (35 %), and in the placebo group, 123 of 268 patients died (46 %). The effect of radium-223 on overall survival was consistent across all subgroups, and radium-223, as compared with placebo, was not associated with significantly more grade 3 or 4 toxic effects.

In the updated analysis, the median overall survival was 14.9 months in the radium-223 group and 11.3 months in the placebo group. The updated analysis confirmed the 30 % reduction in the risk of death among patients in the radium-223 group as compared with the placebo group (hazard ratio, 0.70; 95 % CI, 0.58–0.83; $P < 0.001$). A total of 528 patients in the intention-to-treat population died. In the radium-223 group, 333 of 614 patients died (54 %), and in the placebo group, 195 of 307 patients died (64 %). The effect of radium-223 on overall survival was consistent across all subgroups [82].

In May 2013, the Food and Drug Administration (FDA) approved radium-223 dichloride for the treatment of patients CRPC with symptomatic bone metastases, and no known visceral metastatic disease.

AZD3514: SARD

AZD3514 has a novel mechanism and is able to inhibit AR signaling in androgen-dependent and independent conditions. The compound prevents nuclear transloca-tion of AR and inhibits AR synthesis, with sustained exposure leading to a detect-able downregulation of the receptor.

Because intrinsic or acquired resistance to current antiandrogen therapies is frequently mediated by AR, an inhibitor that also reduces AR levels may conceiv-ably be beneficial in circumventing, or helping to delay the emergence of resis-tance. Such an approach may deliver benefit in CRPC either alone or in combination with other therapies [83].

Interesting is the first-in-human study in which AZD3514 has demonstrated antitumor activity in patients with advanced CRPC: 49 CRPC patients have been treated with escalating doses of AZD3514 (A 35 patients and B 14 patients). The most frequent drug-related AEs were N: G1/2 36/49 (73 %) and G3 2/49 (4 %) and V: G1/2 24/49 (49 %) and G3 3/49 (6 %). N/V were managed with oral antiemetics. Dose proportional increases in plasma concentrations were observed following a single dose. Objective soft tissue responses per RECIST1.1 were observed in 2/26 (8 %) patients. At 6 and 12 months, 21 (43 %) and 8 (16 %) patients remained on study without evidence of bone or soft tissue progression, respectively [84].

10.2.2.10 Bone-Target Therapy

Bone loss associated with ADT clearly causes an increased risk of fractures. In addition, 90 % of patients with CRPC develop bone metastases that can cause a local decrease in bone integrity.

Stimulation of osteoclast activity in patients with hormone refractory prostate cancer is not only focal but also generalized involving mechanisms such secondary hyperparathyroidism, and osteoporosis induced by androgen deprivation [85]. Is recommended for the prevention of skeletal-related events (SREs as pathologic fractures, spinal cord compression, surgery, or RT to bone) the use of zoledronic acid: results of Zoledronic Acid Prostate Cancer Study Group in 122 patients who completed a total of 24 months on study, fewer patients in the 4 mg zoledronic acid group than in the placebo group had at least one SRE (38 % vs. 49 %, difference = −11.0 %, 95 % confidence interval [CI] = −20.2 % to −1.3 %, $P = 0.028$), and the annual incidence of SREs was 0.77 for the 4-mg zoledronic acid group vs. 1.47 for the placebo group ($P = 0.005$). The median time to the first SRE was 488 days for the 4-mg zoledronic acid group vs. 321 days for the placebo group ($P = 0.009$). Compared with placebo, 4 mg of zoledronic acid reduced the ongoing risk of SREs by 36 % (risk ratio = 0.64, 95 % CI = 0.485–0.845, $P = 0.002$). Care must be taken in patients with impaired renal function, and treatment is not recommend for men with baseline creatinine clearance <30 mL/min [86].

Denosumab

Denosumab is a fully humanized monoclonal antibody against RANK ligand. This drug increases by 5.6 % bone mineral density of the lumbar spine as compared with a loss of 1.0 % in the placebo group ($P < 0.001$); denosumab increases the total bone mineral density of hip, femoral neck, and distal third of radius at all time points. Patients who received denosumab had a decreased incidence of new vertebral fractures at 36 months (1.5 % vs. 3.9 % with placebo) (relative risk: 0.38; 95 % confidence interval, 12:19–0.78, $P = 0.006$) [87].

In patients with CRPC and bone metastases, zoledronic acid every 4 weeks or denosumab 120 mg every 4 weeks is recommended to prevent or delay disease-associated SREs. A single large phase III trial in men with bone metastases from CRPC has compared denosumab vs. zoledronic acid. Denosumab was superior on SREs [HR 0.82 (0.71–0.95), $P = 0.0002$], but was associated with an increased risk of hypocalcemia (13 % vs. 6 %). Osteonecrosis of the mandible was seen in both the arms of the trial. There was no difference in OS [88].

10.3 Current Overall Management of CRPC

Several new drugs have been developed over the last years and they are now available in the Oncologist portfolio for the management of CRPC. The main cornerstone of treating CRPC is the need for a continuation of ADT with an LHRH analog. Adding a first-generation antiandrogen (bicalutamide, flutamide, or nilutamide) at progression while on an LHRH analog is a reasonable option even though the expectation of a response from this maneuver is limited. Patients undergone CAB and progressing while on CAB, the peripheral antiandrogen should be discontinued to check for an antiandrogen withdrawal response (AAWD). Subsequent treatment with low-dose steroids—namely dexamethasone 0.5 mg daily—has been reported to effective in bringing down the PSA in some patients, but there are no randomized data regarding OS efficacy. Ketoconazole could be also considered, but the low efficacy rate and poor tolerability limit its application.

Rising PSA only should not be regarded as the only criterion for disease progression, but a combination of radiological (radiological criteria and bony vs. visceral disease), clinical (symptomatic), and biochemical assessment should be performed [89].

CRPC patients with asymptomatic or minimally symptomatic disease and who have not received docetaxel chemotherapy should be offered sipuleucel-T—when there is a life expectancy of at least 6 months—or a first-line hormone manipulation in the form of abiraterone + prednisone. Docetaxel could be a reasonable option in those patients not eligible for abiraterone [89, 90].

Symptomatic chemo-naïve CRPC patients should be offered chemotherapy in the form of 3-weekly docetaxel—this treatment has been proven to not only improve OS but also symptom palliation and quality of life. It should be noted that patients with good performance status are expected to attain the maximum benefit from this treatment. The use of abiraterone—despite not formally tested in symptomatic chemo-naïve CRPC patients—is considered reasonable for those who cannot tolerate or refuse docetaxel. Finally, mitoxantrone can provide a palliative benefit for patients unable to tolerate docetaxel but no OS improvement [89, 90].

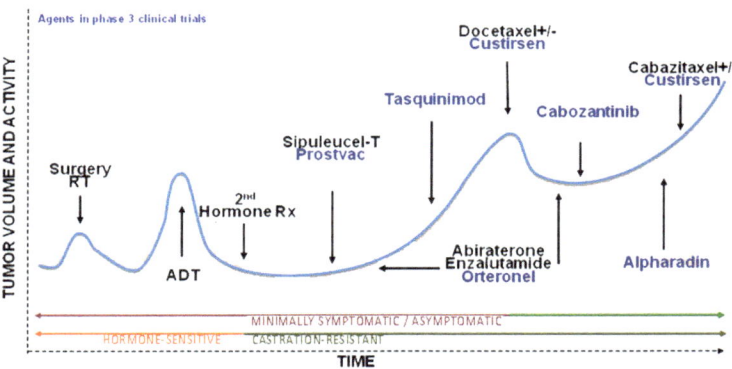

Fig. 10.3 Strategy for optimal squencing for therapeutic agents in metastatic castration resistant prostate cancer. Modified from Zhang et al. [92]

Post-docetaxel CRPC patients not previously exposed to abiraterone and with a good performance status should be offered a further hormone manipulation with abiraterone + prednisone or enzalutamide, but cabazitaxel chemotherapy could be also considered. If the patient has experienced a prolonged progression-free interval after discontinuation of docetaxel, a docetaxel rechallenge could be considered even though there are no phase III trial results supporting this choice [89, 90].

Post-docetaxel CRPC patients with poor performance status have a very limited prognosis and the treatment should aim to improve quality of life [90].

Symptomatic bone metastases can be treated with a systemic treatment (hormonotherapy or chemotherapy) or with a targeted treatment (Radium-223). Single area of painful bony disease as well as spinal cord compression should be treated with radiotherapy. Bisphosphonates or denosumab are used to reduce the incidence of SREs and to improve pain control. Patients with visceral metastasis and symptomatic bone metastases should not be offered a radionuclide treatment as that could preclude further systemic chemotherapy—nevertheless radionuclide treatment could be offered in case the patient is not candidate for further chemotherapy but with the aim of improving the quality of life only [89–91].

In conclusion, treatment of CRPC should be tailored to the patient's characteristics and preference. Dedicated and experienced physicians should be involved in the decision making to optimize the benefit from treatment and minimize the risk of unnecessary toxicity. Disease extent (visceral lesions present or not), performance status, previous treatment(s), symptomatic disease, radiological progression, and biochemical rate of progression should be taken into account before offering a treatment.

One main challenge for the future is to understand the right sequence of treatments nowadays available (Fig. 10.3). A better understanding of molecular biology and discovery of new biomarkers as well as application of new class of drugs in the clinical setting will be crucial to improve outcome of CRPC patients.

References

1. Chen Y, Clegg NJ, Scher HI (2009) Anti-androgens and androgen-depleting therapies in prostate cancer: new agents for an established target. Lancet Oncol 10(10):981–991
2. Holzbeierlein J, Lal P, LaTulippe E et al (2004) Gene expression analysis of human prostate carcinoma during hormonal therapy identifies androgen-responsive genes and mechanisms of therapy resistance. Am J Pathol 164(1):217–227
3. Eisenberger MA, Blumenstein BA, Crawford ED et al (1998) Bilateral orchiectomy with or without flutamide for metastatic prostate cancer. N Engl J Med 339:1036–1042
4. Schmitt B, Bennett C, Seidenfeld J, Samson D, Wilt TJ (1999) Maximal androgen blockade for advanced prostate cancer. Cochrane Database of Syst Rev (2):CD001526. doi:10.1002/14651858.CD001526.5
5. Scher HI, Beer TM, Higano CS et al (2010) Antitumour activity of MDV3100 in castration-resistant prostate cancer: a Phase 1–2 study. Lancet 375(9724):1437–1446. doi:10.1016/S0140-6736 (10) 60172-9
6. Mostaghel EA, Page ST, Lin DW et al (2007) Intraprostatic androgens and androgen-regulated gene expression persist after testosterone suppression: therapeutic implications for castration-resistant prostate cancer. Cancer Res 67(10):5033–5041
7. Bedoya D, Mitsiades N (2012) Abiraterone acetate, a first-in-class CYP17 inhibitor, establishes a new treatment paradigm in castration-resistant prostate cancer. Expert Rev Anticancer Ther 12(1):1–3
8. Logothetis CJ, Gallick GE, Maity SN (2013) Molecular classification of prostate cancer progression: foundation for marker-driven treatment of prostate cancer. Cancer discov 3 (8):849–861. doi:10.1158/2159-8290.CD-12-0460
9. Pfeiffer MJ, Smit FP, Sedelaar JP, Schalken JA (2011) Steroidogenic enzymes and stem cell markers are upregulated during androgen deprivation in prostate cancer. Mol Med 17(7–8):657–664
10. Haapala K, Hyytinen ER, Roiha M, Laurila M et al (2001) Androgen receptor alterations in prostate cancer relapsed during a combined androgen blockade by orchiectomy and bicalutamide. Lab Invest 81:1647–1651
11. Gottlieb B, Beitel LK, Wu JH, Trifiro M (2004) The androgen receptor gene mutations database (ARDB). Hum Mutat 23:527–533
12. Koochekpour S (2010) Androgen receptor signaling and mutations in prostate cancer. Asian J Androl 12(5):639–657. doi:10.1038/aja.2010.89
13. Tran C, Ouk S, Clegg NJ et al (2009) Development of a second-generation antiandrogen for treatment of advanced prostate cancer. Science 324(5928):787–790
14. Tsao C-K, Galsky MD, Small AC et al (2012) Targeting the androgen receptor signalling axis in castration-resistant prostate cancer (CRPC). BJU Int 110(11):1580–1588. doi:10.1111/j.1464-410X.2012.11445.x
15. Kanthoff PW, Halabi S, Conaway M et al (1999) Hydrocortisone with or without mitoxantrone in men with hormone-refractory prostate cancer: results of cancer and leukemia group B 9182 Study. J Clin Oncol 17:2506–2513
16. Tannock IF, Osoba D, Stockler MR et al (1996) Chemotherapy with mitoxantrone plus prednisone or prednisone alone for symptomatic hormone-resistant prostate cancer: a Canadian randomised trial with palliative end points. J Clin Oncol 14:1756–1764
17. Petrylak DP, Tangen CM, Hussain MH et al (2004) Docetaxel and estra-mustine compared with mitoxantrone and prednisone for advanced refractory prostate cancer. N Engl J Med 351:1513–1520
18. Scher HI, Fizazi K, Saad F et al (2012) Increased survival with enzalutamide in prostate cancer after chemotherapy. N Engl J Med 367:1187
19. Tannock IF, de Wit R, Berry WR et al (2004) Docetaxel plus prednisone or mitoxantrone plus prednisone for advanced prostate cancer. N Engl J Med 351:1502–1512

20. Kuroda K, Liu H, Kim S et al (2009) Docetaxel down-regulates the expression of androgen receptor and prostate-specific antigen but not prostate-specific membrane antigen in prostate cancer cell lines: implications for PSA surrogacy. Prostate 69:1579–1585
21. Gan L, Chen S, Wang Y et al (2009) Inhibition of the androgen receptor as a novel mechanism of taxol chemotherapy in prostate cancer. Cancer Res 69:8386
22. Sanofi-Aventis (2010) Jevtana(cabazitaxel) injection prescribing information. Sanofi-Aventis, Bridgewater, NJ
23. Attard G, Greystoke A, Kaye S, de Bono J (2006) Update on tubulin binding agents. Pathol Biol 54:72–84
24. Aller AW, Kraus LA, Bissery MC (2000) In vitro activity of TXD258 in chemotherapeutic resistant tumor cell lines. Proc Am Assoc Cancer Res 41:303, abstr 1923
25. Bissery MC, Bouchard H, Riou JF et al (2000) Preclinical evaluation of TXD258, a new taxoid. Proc Am Assoc Cancer Res 41:214, abstr 1364
26. Oudard S (2011) TROPIC: phase III trial of cabazitaxel for the treatment of metastatic castration-resistant prostate cancer. Future Oncol 7:497–506
27. Bahl A, Oudard S, Tombal B et al (2013) Impact of cabazitaxel on 2-year survival and palliation of tumor-related pain in men with metastatic castration-resistant prostate cancer treated in the TROPIC trial. Ann Oncol 24(9):2402–2408. doi:10.1093/annonc/mdt194
28. de Bono JS, Sartor O (2011) Cabazitaxel for castration-resistant prostate cancer-Authors' reply (letter). Lancet 377:122–123
29. Bahl A, Masson S, Birtle A et al (2013) Second-line treatment options in metastatic castration-resistant prostate cancer: a comparison of key trials with recently approved agents. Cancer Treat Rev 1:170–177. doi:10.1016/j.ctrv.2013.06.008
30. Attard G, Reid AH, Yap TA et al (2008) Phase I clinical trial of a selective inhibitor of CYP17, abiraterone acetate, confirms that castration-resistant prostate cancer commonly remains hormone driven. J Clin Oncol 26(28):4563–4571. doi:10.1200/JCO.2007.15.9749
31. Fizazi K, Scher HI, Molina A et al (2012) Abiraterone acetate for treatment of metastatic castration-resistant prostate cancer: final overall survival analysis of the COU-AA-301 randomised, double-blind, placebo-controlled phase 3 study. Lancet Oncol 13(10):983–992
32. Attard G, Reid AH, A'Hern R et al (2009) Selective inhibition of CYP17 with abir-aterone acetate is highly active in the treatment of castration-resistant prostate cancer. J Clin Oncol 27:3742–3748
33. Ryan CJ, Smith MR, Fong L et al (2010) Phase I clinical trial of the CYP17 inhibitor abiraterone acetate demonstrating clinical activity in patients with castration-resistant prostate cancer who received prior ketoconazole therapy. J Clin Oncol 28:1481–1488
34. Ryan CJ, Shah S, Efstathiou E et al (2011) Phase II study of abiraterone acetate in chemotherapy-naive metastatic castration-resistant prostate cancer displaying bone flare discordant with serologic response. Clin Cancer Res 17:4854–4861
35. Ryan CJ, Smith MR, De Bono JS et al (2012) Interim analysis (IA) results of COU-AA-302, a randomized, phase III study of abiraterone acetate (AA) in chemotherapy-naive patients (pts) with metastatic castration-resistant prostate cancer (mCRPC). Proc Am Soc Clin Oncol 30 (suppl), abstr LBA4518
36. Ryan C (2010) Abiraterone in prostate cancer. Clin Adv Hematol Oncol 8:761–762
37. Sartor O (2011) Combination therapy: abiraterone prolongs survival in metastatic prostate cancer. Nat Rev Clin Oncol 8:515–516
38. Pezaro CJ, Mukherji D, De Bono JS (2012) Abiraterone acetate: redefining hormone treatment for advanced prostate cancer. Drug Discov Today 17(5–6):221–226. doi:10.1016/j.drudis.2011.12.012
39. Handratta VD, Vasaitis TS, Njar VC et al (2005) Novel C- 17-heteroaryl steroidal CYP17 inhibitors/antiandrogens: synthesis, in vitro biological activity, pharmacokinetics, and antitumor activity in the LAPC4 human prostate cancer xenograft model. J Med Chem 48:2972–2984. doi:10.1021/jm040202w

40. Vasaitis T, Belosay A, Schayowitz A et al (2008) Androgen receptor inactivation contributes to antitumor efficacy of 17α-hydroxylase/17,20-lyase inhibitor 3β-hydroxy-17-(1H -benzimidazole-1-yl) androsta-5,16-diene in prostate cancer. Mol Cancer Ther 7:2348–2357. doi:10.1158/1535-7163.MCT-08-0230

41. Montgomery RB, Eisenberger MA, Rettig M et al (2012) Phase I clinical trial of galeterone (TOK-001), a multifunctional antiandrogen and CYP17 inhibitor in castration resistant prostate cancer (CRPC). J Clin Oncol 30(Suppl), abstr 4665

42. Hara T, Kouno J, Kaku T et al (2013) Effect of a novel 17,20-lyase inhibitor, orteronel (TAK-700), on androgen synthesis in male rats. J Steroid Biochem Mol Biol 134:80–91. doi:10.1016/j. jsbmb.2012.10.020

43. Dreicer R, Agus DB, MacVicar GR et al (2010) Safety, pharmacokinetics, and efficacy of TAK-700 in metastatic castration-resistant prostate cancer: a phase I/II, open-label study [abstr 3084]. J Clin Oncol 28(15 suppl):254s

44. Jung ME, Ouk S, Yoo D et al (2010) Structure-activity relationship for thiohydantoin androgen receptor antagonists for castration-resistant prostate cancer (CRPC). J Med Chem 53:2779–2796

45. Rathkopf DE, Morris MJ, Fox JJ et al (2013) Phase I study of ARN-509, a novel antiandrogen, in the treatment of castration-resistant prostate cancer. J Clin Oncol 31(28):3525–3530. doi:10.1200/JCO.2013.50.1684

46. Bianchini D, Zivi A, Sandhu S, De Bono JS (2010) Horizon scanning for novel therapeutics for the treatment of prostate cancer. Ann Oncol 21(Suppl 7):vii43–vii55. doi:10.1093/annonc/mdq369

47. Graddis TJ, McMahan CJ, Tamman J et al (2011) Prostatic acid phosphatase expression in human tissues. Int J Clin Exp Pathol 4(3):295–306

48. Sims RB (2012) Development of sipuleucel-T: autologous cellular immunotherapy for the treatment of metastatic castrate resistant prostate cancer. Vaccine 30(29):4394–4397. doi:10.1016/j.vaccine.2011.11.058

49. Small EJ, Schellhammer PF, Higano CS et al (2006) Placebo-controlled phase III trial of immunologic therapy with sipuleucel-T (APC8015) in patients with metastatic, asymptomatic hormone refractory prostate cancer. J Clin Oncol 24:3089–3094

50. Higano CS, Schellhammer PF, Small EJ (2009) Integrated data from 2 randomized, double-blind, placebo-controlled, phase 3 trials of active cellular immunotherapy with sipuleucel-T in advanced prostate cancer. Cancer 115(16):3670–3679. doi:10.1002/cncr.24429

51. Kantoff PW, Higano CS, Shore ND, IMPACT Study Investigators et al (2010) Sipuleucel-T immunotherapy for castrate-resistant prostate cancer. N Engl J Med 363(5):411–422

52. Plosker GL (2011) Sipuleucel-T: in metastatic castration-resistant prostate cancer. Drugs 71 (1):101–108. doi:10.2165/11206840-000000000-00000

53. Di Paola RS, Plante M, Kaufman H et al (2006) A phase I trial of pox PSA vaccines (PROSTVAC-VF) with B7-1, ICAM-1, and LFA-3 co-stimulatory molecules (TRICOM) in patients with prostate cancer. J Transl Med 4:1

54. DiPaola RS, Chen Y, Bubley GJ et al (2009) A phase II study of PROSTVAC-V (vaccinia)/TRICOM and PROSTVAC-F (fowlpox)/TRICOM with GM-CSF in patients with PSA progression after local therapy for prostate cancer: results of ECOG 9802. In: Genitourinary cancers symposium 2009, abstr 108

55. Kantoff PW, Schuetz TJ, Blumenstein BA et al (2010) Overall survival analysis of a phase II randomized controlled trial of a poxviral-based PSA-targeted immunotherapy in metastatic castration-resistant prostate cancer. J Clin Oncol 28:1099–1105, PubMed: 20100959

56. Gulley JL, Arlen PM, Madan RA et al (2010) Immunologic and prognostic factors associated with overall survival employing a poxviral-based PSA vaccine in metastatic castrate-resistant prostate cancer. Cancer Immunol Immunother 59:663–674, PubMed: 19890632

57. Bilusic M, Gulley J, Heery C et al (2011) A randomized phase II study of flutamide with or without PSA-TRICOM in nonmetastatic castration-resistant prostate cancer (CRPC) [abstr]. J Clin Oncol 29(7S):163

58. Madan RA, Mohebtash M, Arlen PM et al (2010) Overall survival (OS) analysis of a phase 1 trial of a vector-based vaccine (PSA-TRICOM) and ipilimumab (Ipi) in the treatment of metastatic castration-resistant prostate cancer (mCRPC): a double-blinded randomized phase I/II study. In: Program and abstracts of the 2010 American Society of Clinical Oncology Genitourinary Cancers symposium, San Francisco, CA, 5–7 March 2010. Abstract

59. Tollefson MK, Karnes RJ, Thompson RH et al (2010) A randomized phase II study of ipilimumab with androgen ablation compared with androgen ablation alone in patients with advanced prostate cancer. In: Program and abstracts of the 2010 American Society of Clinical Oncology Genitourinary Cancers symposium, San Francisco, CA, 5–7 March 2010, abstr 168

60. Olsson A, Björk A, Vallon-Christersson J et al (2010) Tasquinimod (ABR-215050), a quino-line-3-carboxamide anti-angiogenic agent, modulates the expression of thrombospondin-1 in human prostate tumors. Mol Cancer 9:107

61. Jennbacken K, Welen K, Olsson A et al (2012) Inhibition of metastasis in a castration resistant prostate cancer model by the quinoline-3-carboxamide tasquinimod (ABR-215050). Prostate 72(8):913–924

62. Scher HI, Halabi S, Tannock I, Prostate Cancer Clinical Trials Working Group et al (2008) Design and end points of clinical trials for patients with progressive prostate cancer and castrate levels of testosterone: recommendations of the Prostate Cancer Clinical Trials Working Group. J Clin Oncol 26(7):1148–1159

63. Pili R, Häggman M, Stadler WM et al (2011) Phase II randomized, double-blind, placebo-controlled study of tasquinimod in men with minimally symptomatic metastatic castrate-resistant prostate cancer. J Clin Oncol 29(30):4022–4028

64. Luo FR, Barrett YC, Yang Z et al (2008) Identification and validation of phospho-SRC, a novel and potential pharmacodynamic biomarker for dasatinib (SPRYCEL), a multi-targeted kinase inhibitor. Cancer Chemother Pharmacol 62:1065–1074, PubMed: 18301894

65. Yu EY, Massard C, Gross ME, Carducci MA et al (2011) Once-daily dasatinib: expansion of phase II study evaluating safety and efficacy of dasatinib in patients with metastatic castration-resistant prostate cancer. Urology 77(5):1166–1171. doi:10.1016/j.urology.2011.01.006

66. Araujo JC, Mathew P, Armstrong AJ et al (2012) Dasatinib combined with docetaxel for castration-resistant prostate cancer: results from a phase 1-2 study. Cancer 118(1):63–71. doi:10.1002/cncr.26204

67. Araujo JC Trudel GC, Fred Saad et al (2013) Overall survival (OS) and safety of dasatinib/docetaxel versus docetaxel in patients with metastatic castration-resistant prostate cancer (mCRPC): results from the randomized phase III READY trial. J Clin Oncol 31(suppl 6), abstr LBA8

68. Smith DC, Smith MR, Sweeney C et al (2013) Cabozantinib in patients with advanced prostate cancer: results of a phase II randomized discontinuation trial. J Clin Oncol 31(4):412–419. doi:10.1200/JCO.2012.45.0494

69. Fong PC, Boss DS, Yap TA et al (2009) Inhibition of poly(ADP-ribose) polymerase in tumors from BRCA mutation carriers. N Engl J Med 361(2):123–134. doi:10.1056/NEJMoa0900212

70. Sandhu SK, Schelman WR, Wilding G et al (2013) The poly(ADP-ribose) polymerase inhibitor niraparib (MK4827) in BRCA mutation carriers and patients with sporadic cancer: a phase 1 dose-escalation trial. Lancet Oncol 14(9):882–892. doi:10.1016/S1470-2045(13)70240-7

71. Zellweger T, Miyake H, Cooper S et al (2001) Antitumor activity of antisense clusterin oligonucleotides is improved in vitro and in vivo by incorporation of 2'-O-(2-methoxy)ethyl chemistry. J Pharmacol Exp Ther 298:934–940

72. Saad F, Hotte S, North S et al (2011) Randomized phase II trial of Custirsen (OGX-011) in combination with docetaxel or mitoxantrone as second-line therapy in patients with metastatic castrate-resistant prostate cancer progressing after first-line docetaxel: CUOG trial P-06c. Clin Cancer Res 17(17):5765–5773. doi:10.1158/1078-0432.CCR-11-0859

73. Chi KN, Hotte SJ, Yu EY et al (2010) Randomized phase II study of docetaxel and prednisone with or without OGX-011 in patients with metastatic castration-resistant prostate cancer. J Clin Oncol 28(27):4247–4254. doi:10.1200/JCO.2009.26.8771

74. Lamoureux F, Thomas C, Yin MJ et al (2011) Clusterin inhibition using OGX-011 synergistically enhances Hsp90 inhibitor activity by suppressing the heat shock response in castrate-resistant prostate cancer. Cancer Res 71(17):5838–5849. doi:10.1158/0008-5472.CAN-11-0994

75. Chi K, Yu EY, Ellard S et al (2012) A randomized phase II study of OGX-427 plus prednisone (P) vs. P alone in patients (pts) with metastatic castration resistant prostate cancer (CRPC). Ann Oncol 23, abstr 900PD

76. MacVicar GR, Hussain MH (2013) Emerging therapies in metastatic castration-sensitive and castration-resistant prostate cancer. Curr Opin Oncol 25(3):252–260. doi:10.1097/CCO.0b013e32835ff161

77. Oh WK, Galsky MD, Stadler WM et al (2011) Multicenter phase II trial of the heat shock protein 90 inhibitor, retaspimycin hydrochloride (IPI-504), in patients with castration-resistant prostate cancer. Urology 78(3):626–630. doi:10.1016/j.urology.2011.04.041

78. Heath EI et al (2005) A phase II trial of 17-allylamino-17-demethoxygeldanamycin in patients with hormone-refractory metastatic prostate cancer. Clin Prostate Cancer 4:138–141

79. Heath EI et al (2008) A phase II trial of 17-allylamino-17-demethoxygeldanamycin in patients with hormone-refractory metastatic prostate cancer. Clin Cancer Res 14:7940–7946

80. Bianchini D, Omlin AG, Pezaro CJ et al (2013) First-in-human phase I study of EZN-4176, a locked nucleic acid antisense oligonucleotide (LNA-ASO) to androgen receptor (AR) mRNA in patients with castration-resistant prostate cancer (CRPC). J Clin Oncol 31(suppl), abstr 5052

81. Vapiwala N, Glatstein E (2003) Fighting prostate cancer with radium-223—not your Madame's isotope. N Engl J Med 369(3):276–278

82. Parker C, Nilsson S, Heinrich D et al (2013) Alpha emitter radium-223 and survival in metastatic prostate cancer. N Engl J Med 369(3):213–223. doi:10.1056/NEJMoa1213755

83. Loddick SA, Ross SJ, Andrew GT et al (2013) AZD3514: a small molecule that modulates androgen receptor signaling and function in vitro and in vivo. Mol Cancer Ther 12:1715–1727

84. Omlin AG, Jones RJ, van der Noll R et al (2013) A first-in-human study of the oral selective androgen receptor down-regulating drug (SARD) AZD3514 in patients with castration-resistant prostate cancer (CRPC). J Clin Oncol 31(suppl), abstr 4511

85. Smith MR (2004) The role of bisphosphonates in men with prostate cancer receiving androgen deprivation therapy. Oncology 18:21–25, 85

86. Saad F, Gleason DM, Murray R et al (2004) Long-term efficacy of zoledronic acid for the prevention of skeletal complications in patients with metastatic hormone-refractory prostate cancer. J Natl Cancer Inst 96(11):879–882

87. Smith MR, Egerdie B, Hernández Toriz N et al (2009) Denosumab in men receiving androgen-deprivation therapy for prostate cancer. N Engl J Med 361(8):745–755. doi:10.1056/NEJMoa0809003

88. Fizazi K, Carducci M, Smith M et al (2011) Denosumab versus zoledronic acid for treatment of bone metastases in men with castration-resistant prostate cancer: a randomized, double-blind study. Lancet 377:813–822

89. Cookson MS, Roth BJ, Dahm P et al (2013) Castration-resistant prostate cancer: AUA guideline. J Urol 190(2):429–438. doi:10.1016/j.juro.2013.05.005

90. Mohler JL, Kantoff PW, Armstrong AJ (2013) Prostate cancer, version 1.2014. J Natl Compr Cancr Netw 11(12):1471–1479

91. Horwich A, Parker C, De Reijke T, Kataja V (2013) Prostate cancer: ESMO clinical practice guidelines for diagnosis, treatment and follow-up. Ann Oncol 21:1–9. doi:10.1093/annonc/mdt208

92. Zhang TY, Agarwal N, Sonpavde G (2013) Management of castrate resistant prostate cancer-recent advances and optimal sequence of treatments. Curr Urol Rep 14(3):174–183. doi:10.1007/s11934-013-0322-0

Focal Therapies: MR-Guided High-Intensity Focused Ultrasound

Alessandro Napoli, Carlo Catalano, and Gaia Cartocci

11.1 Introduction

Focal therapy for prostate cancer (PC) is now considered as an emerging alternative to active surveillance for the managements of low-risk prostate cancer with the overall aim of treating only areas of cancer. In fact, the favorable physical interaction between ultrasound (US) waves and biological tissue promises some very interesting and unique therapeutic approaches. High-Intensity Focused Ultrasound (HIFU) represents an innovative technique that may selectively ablate known disease while preserving existing functions. Combining magnetic resonance imaging (MRI) to define the target, to control and monitor the ablation, and an ultrasound transducer that controls and delivers the focused ultrasound beam, Magnetic Resonance guided Focused Ultrasound (MRgFUS) allows a noninvasive approach to the treatment of PC.

11.2 Focal Therapy

PC is recognized as one of the most common cancer in males all over the world [1]. The introduction of prostate-specific antigen (PSA) testing has led to a profound stage migration with a large proportion of men being diagnosed with a low-stage, low-grade cancer that has minimal risk of progression. [2]. D'Amico et al. developed the concept of risk stratification in 1998. This classification system was designed to evaluate the risk of recurrence following localized treatment of prostate cancer. It categorizes patients into three risk-based recurrence groups: low, intermediate, and high risk, using such measures as blood PSA levels, Gleason grades, and tumor stages via T-scores [3] (Table 11.1). Treatment options for PC

A. Napoli (✉) • C. Catalano • G. Cartocci
Department of Radiological, Pathological and Oncological Sciences, Sapienza University of Rome, Viale Regina 324, 00100 Rome, Italy
e-mail: alessandro.napoli@uniroma1.it

V. Gentile et al. (eds.), *Multidisciplinary Management of Prostate Cancer*,
DOI 10.1007/978-3-319-04385-2_11, © Springer International Publishing Switzerland 2014

Table 11.1 The classification developed by D'Amico and colleagues is one of the most widely used in clinical practice and is a good starting point for risk assessment

Risk classification	Stage	PSA	Gleason
Low risk	T1-2a	≤10 ng/ml	≤6
Intermediated risk	T2b	>10 and ≤ 20 ng/ml	7
High risk	T2c-3a	>20 ng/ml	≥ 8

This system uses PSA level, Gleason grade, and T stage to group men as low, intermediate, or high risk

demonstrate a large spectrum of choices and the management of men with this diagnosis is set to become one of the most challenging public health issues. The problems include overdiagnosis, overtreatment, treatment-related toxicity and escalating, and unsustainable costs [4]. The American Urological Association recommends active surveillance, interstitial prostate brachytherapy, external beam radiation therapy (EBRT) and radical prostatectomy (RP) as therapy option for patients with PC [5]. On the other hand, the European Association of Urology (EAU) guidelines recommend RP for intermediate and high-risk populations. Active surveillance is recommended for the low-risk population, but the patient needs to be informed of risks and other therapy options [6]. Several randomized trial that compared retropubic (RP) to "watchful waiting" showed that RP reduced PC mortality and the risk of metastases [7, 8]. Other studies demonstrated that low-risk prostatic tumors are correlated with a better prognosis in terms of biochemical-free survival and metastatic-free disease [9]. Standard treatment for PC has long been "whole-gland" therapy including RP (i.e., complete surgical removal of the prostate) or radiation therapy of the entire prostate (via external beam or brachytherapy). When we do use radical treatments, such as radiotherapy or surgery, those treatments are directed at the entire organ, because we are not able to accurately localize tumors within the prostate. Whole-gland therapies are prone for damaging neighboring structures such as the bladder neck, external urinary sphincter, neurovascular bundles, and rectum [10]. Such damage can result in significant urinary incontinence requiring pads, erectile dysfunction, and rectal toxicity (proctitis, bleeding, and diarrhea). More recently, there is an increasing interest in alternative strategies and treatment options that lies between active surveillance and radical therapy because several studies demonstrate that small localized well-differentiated tumors will not progress, and radical therapy may lead to substantial overtreatment with resulting effects on the patients' quality of life and treatments costs [11].

The aim of focal therapy is to treat cancer within the prostate, whilst leaving benign prostate and surrounding normal structures intact, in order to offer oncological control with minimum impact on genitourinary and rectal function. This concept is not forgetting the multifocal nature of PC but is based on the assumption that only the index lesion is eventually responsible for severe consequences for patients' life; the remaining lesions are over-treated as they could be successfully managed conservatively. As a consequence, a variety of focal therapies have been proposed and are under clinical evaluation (Laser, CryoAblation, etc.). High-Intensity Focused Ultrasound (HIFU) is emerging as an alternative to active surveillance for the management of low risk of prostate cancer, noninvasively. It represents an innovative technique that may selectively ablate known disease while preserving existing functions [12]. The favorable physical interaction between ultrasound (US) waves and biological tissue promises some very interesting and unique therapeutic approaches. In fact, the conservative approach (sparing also the neurovascular bundle) leads to a low rate of genitourinary side effects. HIFU features high energy ultrasound focused to thermally ablate target tissue by raising the local temperature over 60 °C, leading to coagulative necrosis [13]. First HIFU ablation of PC have been performed under conventional ultrasound (US) guidance [12, 14, 15] more than 15 years ago; at present, HIFU has been presented as an alternative therapeutic options for localized PC in the Guidelines of American Urological Association (AUA) in 2007 [5] and of European Association of Urology (EAU) in 2008 [16]. Recently, Magnetic Resonance Imaging (MRI) has been proposed as a guidance and monitoring modality (Magnetic Resonance guided Focused Ultrasound Surgery—MRgFUS) [17], introducing some relevant advantages over other imaging options, especially superior anatomical resolution and tumor detection, thanks to dynamic contrast enhanced imaging (DCE-MRI), spectroscopy, Diffusion-Weighted Imaging (DWI) [18–20], and fast thermal mapping with the proton-frequency shift (PRF) method, to control temperature rising and confirm ablation in real time during the treatment[21]. MRI can be also performed as posttreatment monitoring technique for immediate evaluation of procedure efficacy [22, 23].

11.3 Focused Ultrasound Principles

High-intensity focused ultrasound therapy is a novel, emerging, therapeutic modality that uses ultrasound waves, propagated through tissue media, as carriers of energy. This completely noninvasive technology has great potential for tumor ablation as well as hemostasis, thrombolysis, and targeted drug/gene delivery [24]. Ultrasound is a pressure wave with a frequency above the audible range of a human ear (18–20 kHz); it is generated by a mechanical motion that induces the molecules in a medium to oscillate around their rest positions. The motion causes compressions and rarefactions of the medium and thus a pressure wave travels with the mechanical disturbance. As a result, an ultrasound wave requires a medium for propagation. Ultrasound is generated by applying radiofrequency (RF) voltage across a material that is piezoelectric, i.e., it expands and contracts in proportion to the applied voltage. For many applications of ultrasound therapy, transducers capable of producing high-power, single-frequency, and continuous waves are needed. In order to be able to use ultrasound for therapy, it is essential to know the ultrasonic properties of tissues. The temperature elevation induced at the focus is partially dependent on the ultrasound attenuation, while the beam propagates through the overlying tissues, and the tissue absorption coefficient at the target site. The speed of ultrasound is not frequency dependent and has a similar average magnitude of 1,550 m/s in all soft tissues (excluding lung). The velocity in fatty tissues is less than that in other soft tissues, being about 1,480 m/s while in the lungs the air spaces reduce the velocity to about 600 m/s. The highest values have been measured in bones, between 1,800 and 3,700 m/s depending on the density, structure, and frequency of the wave. The effect of the temperature-dependent sound speed is small on the field shape and can be ignored when sharply focused fields are used. Ultrasonic attenuation in tissues is a sum of the losses due to absorption and scattering, and it determines the penetration of the beam into the tissue. Ultrasound interacts with tissue through the particle motion and pressure variation associated with wave propagation. First, all ultrasound waves are continuously losing energy through absorption resulting in an increase in temperature within the tissue. If the temperature elevation is large enough and is maintained for an adequate period, the exposure causes tissue damage. This thermal effect that can be used for tissue coagulation or ablation is similar to that obtained using other heating methods with equal thermal exposure. Second, at high-pressure amplitudes, the pressure wave can cause formation of small gas bubbles that concentrate acoustic energy. This type of interaction between a sound wave and a gas body is called cavitation and it can cause a multitude of bioeffects from cell membrane permeability changes to complete destruction of tissue. Finally, the mechanical stress and strain associated with wave propagation may sometimes cause direct changes in a biological system. The thermal effects produced by ultrasound have been utilized in hyperthermia as a cancer therapy as well as in many ultrasound surgery applications. In order to induce thermal tissue damage, the exposure at a given temperature has to exceed a threshold time below which the tissue recovers. The thermal damage threshold depends among other things on tissue type and physiological factors (pH and O_2). The temperature elevation in a tissue depends on the absorption and attenuation coefficients of the tissue, the size and shape of the ultrasound field (thermal conduction effects), and also strongly on the local blood perfusion rate. For HIFU ablation, a piezoelectric transducer with a typical center frequency of between 1 and 7 MHz is used to generate a focused ultrasound field. This field is coupled into the body and aimed at the target region. By propagation through the tissue, the US wave will be absorbed and the acoustic energy will be transformed to heat. Inside the focal zone the high energy density will cause temperature increases to more than 60 °C within seconds, and the tissue proteins to coagulate. The surrounding tissue and the overlying structures remain unaffected due to the low acoustic energy density in this area [15] (Fig. 11.1). Combining MR imaging to define the target and to control and monitor the ablation, and an ultrasound transducer that controls and delivers the focused ultrasound beam, MRgFUS allows a noninvasive approach to the treatment of many malignant or not pathologies. At present, MRI is one of the most accurate techniques to investigate local anatomy of male pelvis in detail and is particularly helpful for localization and staging of PC. Traditional prostate MRI has been based on morphologic imaging with standard T1-weighted and T2-weighted sequences, which has limited

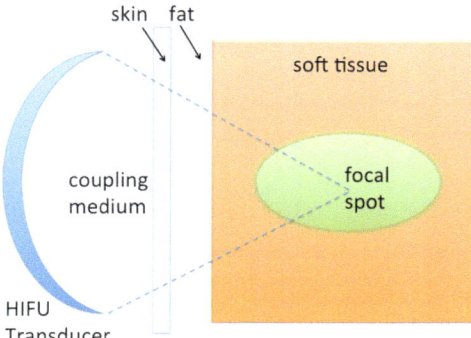

Fig. 11.1 Schematic representation of piezoelectric transducer used to generate a focused ultrasound field. The US wave is absorbed and the acoustic energy is transformed to heat in the focal zone, that rise in temperature over 60 °C. The surrounding tissue and the overlying structures remain unaffected thanks to the low acoustic energy density in this area

accuracy. Recent advances including DWI and perfusion imaging allow extension of the obtainable information beyond anatomic assessment [18]. All these techniques have shown their potential value in distinguishing malignant from benign PC; however, none of them used alone is capable of optimally characterizing tumors in the prostate [25]. For guiding and monitoring HIFU ablation, MRI could be considered more accurate than US as it offers clear advantages: first, it provides high-resolution imaging in any orientation for planning treatment and evaluating relative effects thanks to soft tissue contrast; second, MRI is the only currently available technique with proven capabilities to create quantitative temperature maps. MR-based thermal imaging provides a means to ensure that the proper ultrasound exposures are being applied for a safe and effective ablation on the target volume without effects to surrounding tissues [23, 26]. Magnetic resonance PRF thermometry allows noninvasive temperature monitoring during ultrasound thermal ablation. The method uses the temperature dependence of the PRF which can be determined from the phase in gradient echo images [26, 27]. In order to provide volumetric and rapid thermometry, the acquisition sequences are multislice, gradient-recalled, single-shot, echo-planar imaging (EPI). Moreover, developments in MR imaging hardware and software (3-T vs. 1.5-T imaging) continue to improve spatial and temporal resolution and the signal-to-noise ratio of MR imaging examinations [19].

11.4 MRgFUS: Our Experience

After the wide experience obtained with US-guided HIFU all over the world in the last 15 years, MRgFUS has been successfully tested in small patients groups for the focal therapy of prostate cancer in the last years. At present, in our Department, six patients with unifocal, biopsy proven PC, indicated to RP, underwent MRgFUS

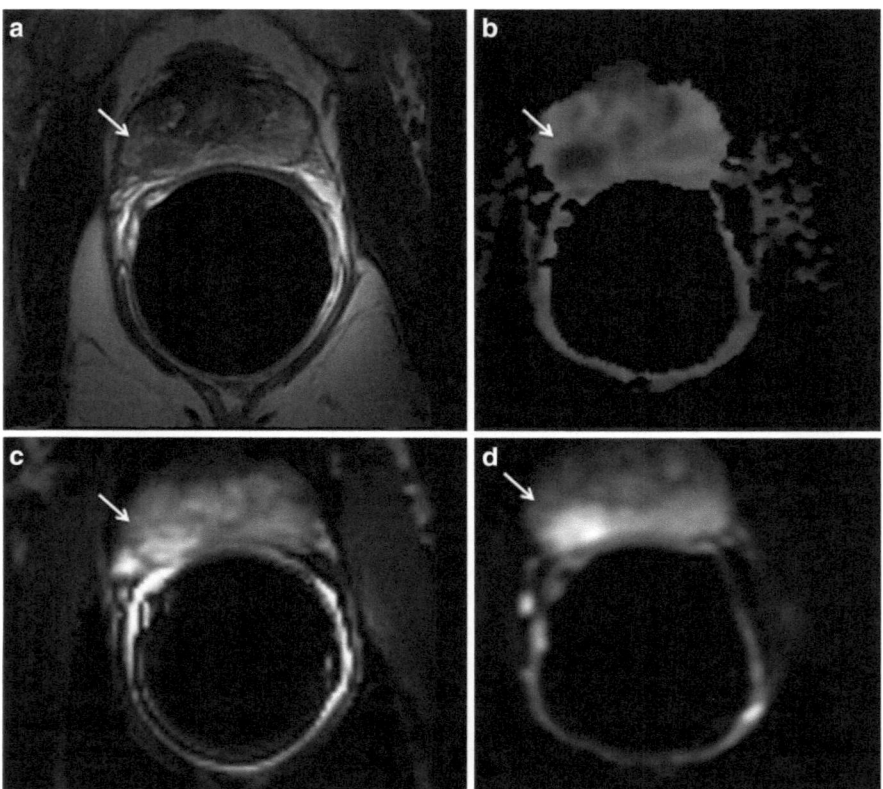

Fig. 11.2 MR imaging of prostate in a 65-year-old man with a focal neoplastic lesion, involving the right peripheral zone (*arrow*). Axial T2-weighted MR image shows a focal low-signal-intensity lesion (**a**); diffusion-weighted imaging (DWI) and correlated ADC map show a focus of restricted diffusion (**b, c**); perfusion weighted imaging (PWI) dynamic sequences show homogenous perfusion of target lesion after administration of contrast medium

prior to surgery in a phase I, controlled trial. All patients included in this study had localized disease (stage T1–T2, Nx–N0, M0), Gleason score 6 (3 + 3), PSA level less than 10 ng/ml, and evidence of cancer lesions on MRI. Target lesions were identified with Turbo Spin Echo T2-weighted, DCE T1-weighted, and DWI sequences and served as planning for subsequent MRgFUS ablation (Fig. 11.2). Patients with a Gleason score ≥8, multifocal or bilateral prostate cancer, with a previous pelvic or rectal cancer, and with an American anesthesiological (ASA) score ≥3 were excluded from the study. All subjects underwent MRgFUS treatment and a subsequent open radical prostatectomy within 2 weeks.

All treatments were performed with an endorectal focused ultrasound ablation system integrated within a 3 T MR scanner (Fig. 11.3). Patients were positioned supine on the scanner table under spinal anesthesia and a 16 F Foley catheter was

Fig. 11.3 Treatments were performed with an endorectal focused ultrasound ablation system (**a**) integrated within a 3T MR scanner (**b**)

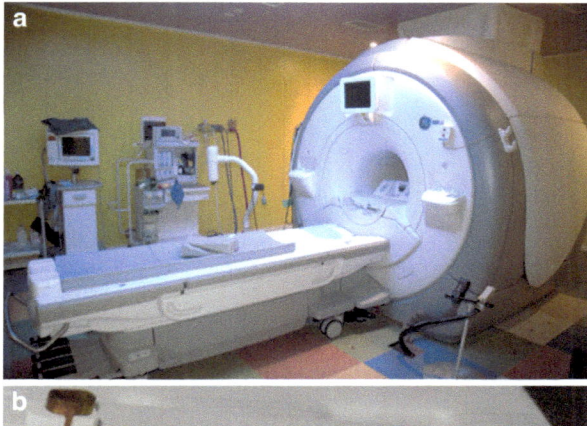

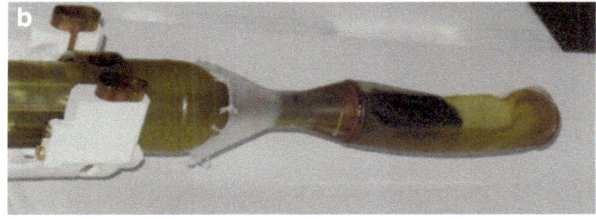

used to ensure urine flow during the procedure. The endorectal probe, which contains a 990-element phased-array focused ultrasound, was inserted into the rectum and filled with degassed water to eliminate residual air within the interface between the prostate and the rectal wall. MRI scan protocol included turbo spin-echo T2-weighted, dynamic contrast-enhanced T1-weighted and Diffusion-weighted sequences in order to correctly localize the target lesion and to allow precise three-dimensional ablation planning. Once the ablation area was identified and manually contoured including 5-mm tumor-free margins, the system generated a patient-specific treatment plan optimizing the required energy level and number of sonications in order to avoid damage to nontargeted tissue and minimize treatment duration. Targeting was confirmed using low-power subtherapeutic sonications monitored with PRF shift method for MRI thermometry, overlapping temperature maps onto anatomic images. After confirmation, treatment started using full-energy sonications in the target area and monitoring in real time each sonication with dedicated MRI sequences for precise temperature mapping. Sonicated volumes were considered successfully ablated when the temperature in the target area reached a threshold of 65 °C. Treatment was considered complete once the lesion and tumor-free margins have been completely ablated and evident as a nonperfused area at MRI (Fig. 11.4). After treatment patients were examined and monitored for adverse events for 3 h prior to discharge, with uneventful course in all cases. The following day all patients received corticosteroids to control local inflammatory reaction. Results of MRgFUS treatment was assessed by a Pathologist comparing the extent of tissue necrosis with histopathology findings after radical surgery of the gland specimen regions of interest were fixed in formalin.

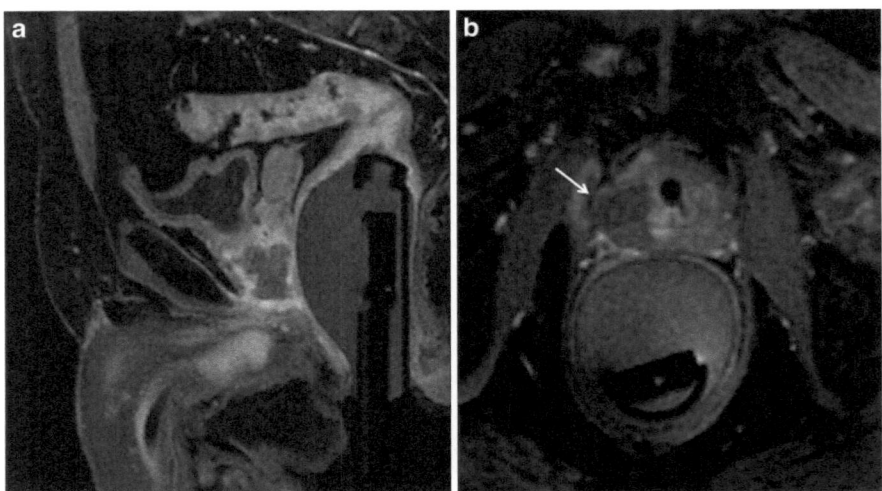

Fig. 11.4 Sagittal (**a**) and axial (**b**) T1-weighted images demonstrate the complete ablation of target lesion as a non-perfused tissue area after administration of contrast medium

No technical difficulties related to MRgFUS ablation or severe complications were encountered during surgery. Standard hematoxylin–eosin (H–E) staining was performed in all the specimens. In all cases, the analysis of the whole prostate section specimens demonstrated extensive coagulative necrosis at the site of sonication surrounded by normal prostatic tissue with inflammatory changes. No residual viable tumor tissue was evidenced in the ablation area or along the safety margins. Our experience showed as MRgFUS can be safely used to identify and treat the target lesion, with no significant side effects and with reproducible results. So far, we planned to evaluate its possible role for the management of patients with localized prostate cancer. Focal therapy of discrete areas of cancer, whether unifocal or multifocal, is feasible, safe, and can be delivered in an ambulatory care setting. Early self-resolving lower urinary-tract symptoms were common. However, the strategy was well tolerated in the genitourinary functional domains. Furthermore, MRgFUS treatment does not impact on the morbidity and oncological outcome of a subsequent radical prostatectomy which was safely performed in all patients. Focal therapy is an attractive alternative option in the management of low-risk prostate cancer. The currently accepted curative treatment approaches for localized prostate cancer depend on patient and tumor factors and account for radical prostatectomy, Radiotherapy/Brachytherapy, and more recently HIFU. The decision to use HIFU rather than surgery is often made on the basis of patient factors. The increased popularity of HIFU relies on many factors; it appears highly attractive as a minimally invasive treatment for localized prostate cancer as HIFU entails no incision or puncture, it is bloodless, can be carried out on an outpatient basis and is repeatable. The clinical outcome of HIFU treatment has significantly improved over the years as a result of technical, imaging, and device improvements; among these improvements, MR guidance is the most advanced that was lastly introduced and has potential to drive this application for a safer and more effective treatment thanks to its superior anatomic resolution and for its capability to perform real-time temperature mapping. Despite initial results on human for feasibility and safety appear highly promising, MRgFUS is still under investigation and more studies are needed to demonstrate the oncologic effectiveness as well as to validate its durable effect on patient outcomes [28].

References

1. Siegel R, Naishadham D, Jemal A (2012) Cancer statistics, 2012. CA Cancer J Clin 62(1): 10–29
2. Singer EA, Kaushal A, Turkbey B, Couvillon A, Pinto PA, Parnes HL (2012) Active surveillance for prostate cancer: past, present and future. Curr Opin Oncol 24(3):243–250
3. Hernandez DJ, Nielsen ME, Han M, Partin AW (2007) Contemporary evaluation of the D'amico risk classification of prostate cancer. Urology 70(5):931–935
4. Ahmed HU, Akin O, Coleman JA, Crane S, Emberton M, Goldenberg L, Hricak H, Kattan MW, Kurhanewicz J, Moore CM et al (2012) Transatlantic Consensus Group on active surveillance and focal therapy for prostate cancer. BJU Int 109(11):1636–1647
5. Thompson I, Thrasher JB, Aus G, Burnett AL, Canby-Hagino ED, Cookson MS, D'Amico AV, Dmochowski RR, Eton DT, Forman JD et al (2007) Guideline for the management of clinically localized prostate cancer: 2007 update. J Urol 177(6):2106–2131
6. Heidenreich A, Abrahamsson PA, Artibani W, Catto J, Montorsi F, Van Poppel H, Wirth M, Mottet N (2013) Early detection of prostate cancer: European Association of Urology recommendation. Eur Urol 64(3):347–354
7. Bill-Axelson A, Holmberg L, Filen F, Ruutu M, Garmo H, Busch C, Nordling S, Haggman M, Andersson SO, Bratell S et al (2008) Radical prostatectomy versus watchful waiting in localized prostate cancer: the Scandinavian prostate cancer group-4 randomized trial. J Natl Cancer Inst 100(16):1144–1154
8. Albertsen P (2009) Words of wisdom. Re: Radical prostatectomy versus watchful waiting in localized prostate cancer: the Scandinavian Prostate Cancer Group-4 randomized trial. Eur Urol 55(4):989–990
9. Klotz L (2008) Active surveillance for prostate cancer: trials and tribulations. World J Urol 26 (5):437–442
10. Wilt TJ, Brawer MK, Jones KM, Barry MJ, Aronson WJ, Fox S, Gingrich JR, Wei JT, Gilhooly P, Grob BM et al (2012) Radical prostatectomy versus observation for localized prostate cancer. N Engl J Med 367(3):203–213
11. Choo R, Klotz L, Danjoux C, Morton GC, DeBoer G, Szumacher E, Fleshner N, Bunting P, Hruby G (2002) Feasibility study: watchful waiting for localized low to intermediate grade prostate carcinoma with selective delayed intervention based on prostate specific antigen, histological and/or clinical progression. J Urol 167(4):1664–1669
12. Maestroni U, Dinale F, Minari R, Salsi P, Ziglioli F (2012) High-intensity focused ultrasound for prostate cancer: long-term follow up and complications rate. Adv Urol 2012:960835
13. Crouzet S, Poissonnier L, Murat FJ, Pasticier G, Rouviere O, Mege-Lechevallier F, Chapelon JY, Martin X, Gelet A (2011) [Outcomes of HIFU for localised prostate cancer using the Ablatherm Integrate Imaging(R) device]. Prog Urol 21(3):191–197
14. Blana A, Rogenhofer S, Ganzer R, Lunz JC, Schostak M, Wieland WF, Walter B (2008) Eight years' experience with high-intensity focused ultrasonography for treatment of localized prostate cancer. Urology 72(6):1329–1333, discussion 1333–1334

15. Jenne JW, Preusser T, Gunther M (2012) High-intensity focused ultrasound: principles, therapy guidance, simulations and applications. Z Med Phys 22(4):311–322
16. Heidenreich A, Bellmunt J, Bolla M, Joniau S, Mason M, Matveev V, Mottet N, Schmid HP, van der Kwast T, Wiegel T et al (2011) EAU guidelines on prostate cancer. Part 1: screening, diagnosis, and treatment of clinically localised disease. Eur Urol 59(1):61–71
17. Jolesz FA (2009) MRI-guided focused ultrasound surgery. Annu Rev Med 60:417–430
18. Vargas HA, Akin O, Franiel T, Mazaheri Y, Zheng J, Moskowitz C, Udo K, Eastham J, Hricak H (2011) Diffusion-weighted endorectal MR imaging at 3 T for prostate cancer: tumor detection and assessment of aggressiveness. Radiology 259(3):775–784
19. Bonekamp D, Jacobs MA, El-Khouli R, Stoianovici D, Macura KJ (2011) Advancements in MR imaging of the prostate: from diagnosis to interventions. Radiographics 31(3):677–703
20. Hoeks CM, Barentsz JO, Hambrock T, Yakar D, Somford DM, Heijmink SW, Scheenen TW, Vos PC, Huisman H, van Oort IM et al (2011) Prostate cancer: multiparametric MR imaging for detection, localization, and staging. Radiology 261(1):46–66
21. Pilatou MC, Stewart EA, Maier SE, Fennessy FM, Hynynen K, Tempany CM, McDannold N (2009) MRI-based thermal dosimetry and diffusion-weighted imaging of MRI-guided focused ultrasound thermal ablation of uterine fibroids. J Magn Reson Imaging 29(2):404–411
22. Kirkham AP, Emberton M, Hoh IM, Illing RO, Freeman AA, Allen C (2008) MR imaging of prostate after treatment with high-intensity focused ultrasound. Radiology 246(3):833–844
23. Quesson B, Laurent C, Maclair G, de Senneville BD, Mougenot C, Ries M, Carteret T, Rullier A, Moonen CT (2011) Real-time volumetric MRI thermometry of focused ultrasound ablation in vivo: a feasibility study in pig liver and kidney. NMR Biomed 24(2):145–153
24. Al-Bataineh O, Jenne J, Huber P (2012) Clinical and future applications of high intensity focused ultrasound in cancer. Cancer Treat Rev 38(5):346–353
25. Delongchamps NB, Rouanne M, Flam T, Beuvon F, Liberatore M, Zerbib M, Cornud F (2011) Multiparametric magnetic resonance imaging for the detection and localization of prostate cancer: combination of T2-weighted, dynamic contrast-enhanced and diffusion-weighted imaging. BJU Int 107(9):1411–1418
26. Kim YS, Trillaud H, Rhim H, Lim HK, Mali W, Voogt M, Barkhausen J, Eckey T, Kohler MO, Keserci B et al (2012) MR thermometry analysis of sonication accuracy and safety margin of volumetric MR imaging-guided high-intensity focused ultrasound ablation of symptomatic uterine fibroids. Radiology 265(2):627–637
27. Yuan J, Mei CS, Panych LP, McDannold NJ, Madore B (2012) Towards fast and accurate temperature mapping with proton resonance frequency-based MR thermometry. Quant Imaging Med Surg 2(1):21–32
28. Napoli A, Anzidei M, De Nunzio C, Cartocci G, Panebianco V, De Dominicis C, Catalano C, Petrucci F, Leonardo C (2012) Real-time magnetic resonance-guided high-intensity focused ultrasound focal therapy for localised prostate cancer: preliminary experience. Eur Urol 63(2): 395–398